SECRET POWER
OF TANTRIK
BREATHING

SECRET POWER OF TANTRIK BREATHING

Techniques for Attaining Health, Harmony, and Liberation

Swami Sivapriyananda

Destiny Books
Rochester, Vermont

Destiny Books
One Park Street
Rochester, Vermont 05767
www.DestinyBooks.com

Destiny Books is a division of Inner Traditions International

Originally published in India in 1983 by Abhinav Publications under the
    title *Secret Power of Tantrik Breathing*
Revised edition published in 1996 by Abhinav Publications
Third edition published in 2005 by Abhinav Publications
First U.S. edition published in 2009 by Destiny Books under the title
    *Secret Power of Tantrik Breathing: Techniques for Attaining Health,
    Harmony, and Liberation*

Library of Congress Cataloging-in-Publication Data
Sivapriyananda, Swami, 1939–1997.
  Secret power of tantrik breathing : techniques for attaining health,
harmony, and liberation / Swami Sivapriyananda.
      p. cm.
  Originally published: New Delhi : Abhinav Publications, c1983.
  Includes bibliographical references and index.
  ISBN 978-1-59477-289-4 (pbk.)
  1. Prânayâma. 2. Tantrism. I. Title.
  RA781.7.S63 2009
  613'.192—dc22

                                                        2009006515

Printed and bound in the United States by the P. A. Hutchison Company

10 9 8 7 6 5 4 3 2 1

Text design and layout by Priscilla Baker
This book was typeset in Garamond Premier Pro and Legacy Sans with
Charlemagne used as a display typeface

CONTENTS

One
AN INTRODUCTION TO TANTRIK BREATHING

Two
SVARODAYA SHASTRA

Three
SVARODAYA SHASTRA AND
HUMAN DESTINY

Four
TANTRIK AND YOGIC PRACTICES
FOR LIBERATION

Chapter One

AN INTRODUCTION TO TANTRIK BREATHING

*T*he act of normal breathing or respiration involves the taking in or inhaling of oxygen-rich air from the environment into the lungs and breathing out or exhaling air laden with carbon dioxide. Air is inhaled when the muscular wall called the diaphragm and the intercostal muscles between the ribs enlarge the chest cavity by expanding outward. This expansion creates a slight vacuum in the lungs and air is sucked in to fill it. The air that enters the body through the two nostrils passes through the pharyngeal tube into the trachea, the main airway. The trachea divides into two bronchi, which in turn divide and branch into bronchioles leading to the alveolar ducts and sacs where the blood-gas exchange takes place. Exhalation is, on the other hand, a passive act and requires no effort. The elastic diaphragm recoils back to its original position and deflates the lungs, pushing the inhaled air out.

Under normal conditions of quiet breathing, all this takes between four to six seconds. Generally, breathing is an automatic process that goes on at the rate of ten to fifteen breaths every minute, without our having to pay conscious attention to it. This automatic nature of breathing is essential to our survival, as each and every cell in our body needs to be constantly supplied with oxygen. The brain cells are especially sensitive and—if starved of oxygen even for a few minutes—they die, never to be replaced again.

Breathing, however, is not always automatic: unlike the heartbeat and processes of digestion, we can override the respiratory center in the brain and hold our breath. "Respiratory center" is the collective name for the group of brain cells that govern respiration. They are situated at the back of the brain in the region known as the medulla oblongata. As this center has nerve connections to the higher centers of the brain and spinal cord, the emotional states of our mind profoundly influence breathing. Emotional stress can increase the rate of respiration, while emotional calm makes the breathing deep and slow.

The intimate relationship between respiration and the changing emotional states of the mind was known to human beings long before the birth of modern science. Most early civilizations, and particularly those of India and China, evolved methods of controlling respiration and consequently changing the emotions and the state of consciousness.

Very fast and deep breathing over long periods results in too quick a loss of carbon dioxide. This leads to muscle rigidity, stupor, and cataleptic coma. Conversely, a rise in the level of carbon dioxide decreases the oxygen content, which results in anoxia, a feeling of lightheadedness, and a trancelike state in which subjects occasionally have mystical experiences. Many religions use prolonged chanting, shouting, singing, and dancing to induce trancelike states, by increasing the carbon dioxide content of the blood. Another method for doing this is slow breathing.

In India these practices and the theories behind them have been extensively developed in the traditional spiritual disciplines of Tantra and Yoga. The central focus of the Tantra philosophy is the universal energy and creative power represented by the feminine aspect of the Supreme (personified as Shakti or Prakriti or other feminine deities). The tantrik texts contain material that develops the five themes of creation, dissolution, worship, supernatural attainments (*siddhis*), and methods of attaining union with the Supreme through meditation. Yoga seeks union with the Supreme through an eight-fold path (*ashtanga yoga*).

These tantrik and yogic ideas and practices form the background of the tantrik breathing method presented in this book, which is known as *svara-udaya,* or *svarodaya*. The vital breath is called *svara,* and the movement of this svara from nostril to nostril is called *udaya* (rise). The ancient and occult system of knowledge (*shastra*) that deals with the significance of the changes in vital breath is called the svara-udaya or *svarodaya shastra*.

The principles of Tantra, Yoga, svarodaya shastra, and other traditional spiritual disciplines operate entirely on the subtle level, based on principles that may seem a little strange to the modern mind. This is understandable. The demands of daily living today are so great on the outer and practical side of our personality that we have no time to even consider the possibility that there might be an inner, subtle side to our nature. As we have lost contact with the subtle mind, we do not understand the rules governing the hidden and subtle aspect of ourselves. However, recent scientific experiments and tests of yogis and mystics have proved what theories of brain function once held to be impossible: they were able to bring automatic body mechanisms under voluntary mind control. As a result of such studies, many doctors and scientists now agree that the secret of these yogic skills lies in techniques of meditation and the yogic method known as *pranayama,* which both attempt to regulate the carbon dioxide and oxygen ratio of the blood in order to induce mystical states. The details of pranayama principles and practice provide an essential background for understanding the svarodaya method.[1]

Pranayama

The word *pranayama* is composed of two words: *prana,* which means "breath," as well as the vital energies of the human body, and *ayama,* which means "conscious control." Together the words refer to the method of breath control that forms one of the eight basic steps of the classical science of yoga.

All yogic practices start with *yama,* which is concerned ①
with moral discipline and is achieved by taking vows of non-injury, truthfulness, honesty, continence, noncovetousness, forgiveness, pure diet, and cleanliness. Then comes *niyama,* ②
which is moral discipline at a more subtle level and involves internal purity, contentment, austerity, spiritual study, and self surrender. *Asana* is the third stage—physical postures ③
that help to keep the body healthy so that it is possible to sit in meditation for long hours without discomfort. Pranayama ④
is the fourth stage and stands on the border between the physical and psychic aspects of yoga. After pranayama comes *pratyahara,* the withdrawal of consciousness from the senses ⑤
and turning it inward for the next stage of *dharana* or men- ⑥
tal concentration. The seventh stage is reached when dharana ⑦
becomes absolutely steady and one-pointed with no disturb-ing thoughts entering the mind. This is called *dhyana,* or ⑧
true meditation. The final stage is *samadhi,* or trance, in which the individual mind is freed from all material limits and is dissolved into the ultimate Reality.

Pranayama has three steps, which are the same as the three acts of natural respiration; they consist of inhalation (*puraka*), retention (*kumbhaka*), and exhalation (*rechaka*) of air from the lungs. The only difference between the two is that in natural respiration the rhythm is constant while in pranayama it is consciously changed to suit the different types of pranayama.

⚭

PRACTICING PRANAYAMA

Pranayama can be done at any time of the day or night. The actual practice of pranayama starts with finding a clean, quiet, and pleasant spot and sitting on a washed cotton cloth or a woolen mat. The yogic texts usually recommend *siddhasana* (adept's posture) or *padmasana* (lotus posture), but any comfortable posture will do, provided the spine is kept erect and the head is held up in line with the spine.

According to the Hatha Yoga Pradipika (I, 35, 44–45) these two postures are formed in the following manner.

Siddhasana

1. Press the left heel against the perineum, and place the right heel above it.
2. Fix the chin on the chest, straighten the spine, and concentrate on the area between the eyebrows.

   This is the siddhasana, giver of freedom from diseases and the cycle of rebirths.

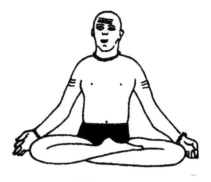

Siddhasana

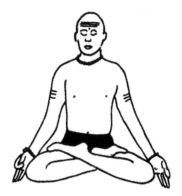

Padmasana

Fig. 1.1. Asanas, or postures, for pranayama

Padmasana

1. Place the right foot at the root of the left thigh and the left foot at the root of the right thigh.

2. Cross the arms behind the back and hold the right toe with the left hand and the left toe with the right hand.*

---

*For meditating in padmasana, it is not necessary to hold the toes; the hands can be kept on the knees.

3. Rest the chin firmly on the chest and fix the sight on the tip of the nose.

This is the padmasana, destroyer of all bodily afflictions.

The Forms of Pranayama

Now practice one of the following forms of pranayama.

1. *Bhastrika:* quick inhalation and exhalation through both the nostrils, which is said to clear the nasal passage and the subtle channels.

2. *Surya bhedana* (conquest of the sun): quick inhalation through the right nostril, then retention and exhalation through the left nostril, which is used to calm the mind.

3. *Ujjayi* (upward restraint): inhalation through both the nostrils and exhalation through the left nostril, which helps to clear all diseases caused by too much phlegm and to strengthen the heart muscles.

4. *Shitali* (cooling): inhalation through the mouth while cupping the tongue and exhalation through both the nostrils, which is said to prolong youth and help digestion.

5. *Plavini* (swimming): long retention after slow inhalation.

6. *Kevala kumbhaka* (simple retention): just retention of breath without any special inhalation or exhalation.

7. *Bhramari* (bee-like): humming during any inhalation is said to clear the throat and the vocal cords.

Blocking Nostrils during Pranayama

When it becomes necessary to block either of the two nostrils during pranayama, the ring and little fingers of the right hand should be used to block the left nostril and the thumb to close the right nostril. The index and middle fingers should never be used. The usual ratio of the three acts of inhalation, retention, and exhalation is 1 : 4 : 2, but this can be changed to suit the particular pranayama.

Chakra Meditation during Pranayama

During inhalation, meditation on the *manipura chakra* (solar plexus) is known to lead the mind quickly into samadhi. Meditation on the *anahata chakra* (cardiac plexus) is recommended during retention and on the *ajna chakra* (optic thalamus) during exhalation. (For the location of these chakras please refer to fig. 1.2 on page 30.)

Pranayama Accompanied by Sound

Pranayama can be either silent (*agarbha*) or accompanied by a *mantra,* or sound pattern (*sagarbha*). Generally, the basic mantra *OM* is used. This is made up of three syllables: *A, U,* and the nasal sound *M*. According to the Dhyana Bindu Upanishad, inhalation is accompanied by the syllable *U,* retention by *M,* and exhalation by *A*.

Besides the change in the oxygen–carbon dioxide ratio of the blood, the yogic method of breath control (pranayama) influences the thought process in another way. It is well known that the normal rate of respiration is related to bodily activity and the emotional state of the individual. Physical exercises and violent emotions such as anger, anxiety, fear, and sexual arousal increase the rate of breathing. A peaceful mind and emotional calm slows down the respiratory rate, sometimes even below the normal level.

Scientists have observed that even among animals, those that are excitable breathe more quickly than those that are placid by nature. A hare breathes 55 times per minute, an ape 30 times, a cat 24 times, a dog 15–18 times, a horse 8–12 times, and a tortoise only 3 times a minute. On the basis of this, yogis argue that if emotional states can affect the rate of breathing, then conversely, an alteration in the rate of respiration should alter the individual's emotional state. All methods of pranayama are based on this basic idea. The final aim of Yoga is to reduce breathing to the absolute minimum, thereby arresting totally the discursive and emotional functions of the mind (*yogah citta vrtti nirodhah*, Patanjala Yogasutra, I, 2).

It is important to remember that no book can teach the practical art of breath control. This can be learned from only a yogi guru. As the Hatha Yoga Pradipika warns:

Pranayama performed correctly destroys all diseases, while incorrectly done pranayama can be the cause of all ills.

When pranayama is done correctly, the mind becomes calm and its processes become subtle. This leads to one-pointedness and concentration. Sensual concerns automatically fall away from a concentrated mind. The mind that is free from outer attractions goes deeper and deeper into meditation until it is totally absorbed into samadhi, the final goal of Yoga.

The Knowledge of the Rise of the Vital Breath (Svarodaya Shastra)

Svarodaya shastra is not a method of breath control but a way of using normal respiration to harmonize the forces of life with the pattern of breathing. The svarodaya technique is based on one basic observable fact that is frequently overlooked. That is, we normally breathe freely through only one nostril at a time. This alternate breathing changes roughly every hour from one nostril to the other.

ॐ

DETERMINING THE OPEN NOSTRIL

It is very easy to find out which channel is open at any given time. Alternately block each nostril for a few seconds. The nostril through which breathing is easy and without strain is the side of the open channel.

There is a qualitative difference between the breath from the left and right nostrils. Breath from the left nostril is cool, soothing, passive, and feminine in nature, while the breath that flows from the right nostril is warm, energizing, active, and masculine. The basic purpose of the svarodaya method is to teach humankind the way of harmonizing the breath from each nostril with the nature of the life task to be accomplished.

Some modern scientific research has been done on the mechanism of alternate nostril dominance while breathing, but no attempt has been made to correlate these nostril changes with certain psychological and behavioral tendencies. Dr. Vijayendra Pratap had ninety-nine people observe nostril activity and record the results for two months (1971–72). They noted the condition of nostril activity each day at 3 hour intervals, from 6 a.m. to 9 p.m. Most of the ninety-nine observers were hospital patients. Statistical analysis of the data collected confirmed variable nostril dominance but could not be used to confirm the rhythmicity of change. Regarding the cause of alternate breathing, Dr. Pratap says:

It is believed that it has something to do with sympathetic innervation. The author of this research paper feels that air currents that pass through the nose stimulate certain parts of the olfactory nerve filaments, and consequently the olfactory bulb, which is an extension of the brain, allowing impulses to continue after a stimulus has ceased. . . . It is possible that central mechanisms govern nostril breathing in order to maintain homeostasis of the organism. . . . It may be surmised that the air currents passing through the right nostril influence *excitatory* effects, while those passing through the other nostril produce *inhibitory* effects.[2]

The significance of nostrils in breathing and the force of breath from each nostril has been scientifically studied by Bhole and Karambelkar (1968). In this study, seventy-seven men and twenty-one women, all in good health, were observed to determine "resting state" breathing patterns. The method of study involved the use of a tube from each nostril, which was attached to a device to record the force of breathing. In 47.8 percent of the cases, the breathing force was greater from the right nostril than the left. In 37.7 percent, the left-nostril breathing force was greater. In only 14.5 percent of the cases was the breathing force of equal magnitude in the right and left nostrils.

According to the svarodaya tradition a particular mode of nostril dominance is preferable for certain activities, and to some extent it is possible to change the breath from one nostril to the other. Tantrik methods of doing this are given in the next chapter. Modern studies to investigate the efficacy of traditional Yoga techniques were conducted by Bhole (1968). He paid special attention to the use of a Y-shaped crutchlike instrument called a *yoga danda* for changing nostril breathing. Subjects were asked to place the yoga danda under an armpit and then lean over and press it between the chest and the arm. This position was maintained for approximately fifteen minutes while the breathing force from each nostril was carefully recorded. Results suggested that the breathing force is increased in the nostril on the side opposite to the yoga danda and decreased in the nostril on the same side.[3]

Rao and Potdar (1970) investigated relative nostril minute ventilation in three horizontal postures. They found that in the supine posture, average minute ventilation was about the same in each nostril. However, for the right lateral posture, with the subjects lying comfortably on a bed with the weight of the body borne on the lateral aspect of the thigh, temporal region, shoulder, and arm, average minute ventilation was greater through the left nostril. It was exactly the opposite of this in the left lateral posture. In short, the "up" nostril was always more active. Rao and Potdar concluded that though the nature of this mechanism was not yet very clear, the variation in blood flow through the nasal mucosa may account for the variations in relative nostril ventilation.[4]

Yoga texts say that if one is successful in gaining control over the change of breath from one nostril to the other and can bring about the change at will without resorting to any physical method, then one is said to be freed from destiny. Some also say that the tossing and turning that we do at night in sleep is nature's way of maintaining the balance of the two forces in the human body.

Shiva Svarodaya Shastra

Traditionally the svarodaya method was first taught by Lord Shiva—the storehouse of all occult knowledge—to his wife Parvati—a personification of his occult power (Shakti). The legend says that Parvati fell asleep while listening to Shiva's hypnotic voice explaining the secrets of the svarodaya technique. But a fisherman, or a shaman who had turned himself into a fish, heard the entire exposition. This shaman was the great occultist Matsyendranatha. He remembered every word Shiva had spoken and he passed the knowledge (*Shiva svarodaya shastra*) to humankind through a long line of disciples known throughout Indian literature and religion as the Nathas (masters).

The word *natha* is very interesting and its mystical etymology is subtly related to the cosmic philosophy of the Natha sect. It has two syllables: *na* and *tha*. *Na* is said to represent the unmanifested cosmic spirit, and *tha* symbolizes the manifested universe. Therefore, a Natha is a person who understands and harmonizes the two polarities of the unmanifest and the manifest.

In order to understand the ancient system of the harmony of breath it is important to comprehend the basic concepts on which this system is based, which include a theory of evolution and the vital energy.

Evolution

The first of these concepts is the evolution of the universe. But it should be clearly understood that this occult theory of evolution does not refer to the physical universe. It represents the gradual awakening of the individual's consciousness. Therefore, it refers to the psychological and psychic universe.

The evolution of this microcosm/macrocosm is the result

of an interaction between the "principle of consciousness" (Purusha) or the positive/male element and the "energy of nature" (Prakriti) or the negative/female element.

In the beginning, the three potentials or qualities of the universe (*gunas*)—luminosity, existence, goodness (*sattva*); activity, movement, motor energy (*rajas*); and sloth, static inertia, darkness (*tamas*)—lay in perfect and homogeneous balance within Prakriti. Then, in time (*kala*), the proximity of the Purusha to the Prakriti upset the perfect primordial equilibrium and the process of evolution was set in motion. From the transformations that took place within the Prakriti principle, the essence of intellect and the foundation of all mental functions (*buddhi* or *mahat*) was born (see plate 1 for a traditional symbolic rendering of buddhi). Drawn by the force of evolution, Prakriti was transformed from the state of buddhi to that of *ahamkara*—the sense of I-ness and the basic notion of individual existence (ego).

From ahamkara, evolution proceeded in two directions: the objective or external world and the subjective or psycho-mental world. The evolutionary direction that ahamkara took depended upon which of the three gunas predominated. When sattva, or luminosity, predominated, then the mind (*manas*), five sense organs (*jnana indriyas*)—ears, skin, eyes, tongue, and nose—and the five sense percep-tions—hearing, feeling, seeing, tasting, and smelling—

were evolved. When rajas, or movement, was dominant, the five organs of action (*karma indriyas*)—mouth, hands, legs, bowels, and genitals—and the five basic actions—speaking, grasping, walking, excreting, and copulating—came into being. With the predominance of tamas, or inertia, there appeared the five potential elements (*tanmatras*), their subtle qualities of sound, touch, form, flavor, and odor, and the five gross elements (*mahabhutas*)—space (*akasha*), air (*vayu*), fire (*tejas*), water (*ap*), and earth (*prithvi*) (see the table opposite).

The five gross elements make up the physical world we see around us. But they never exist in their pure state. The actual earth, for instance, is only 50 percent earth and about 12 percent of each of the other four—water, fire, air, and space. All material and visible forms of the five gross elements have a similar composition.

After a set period of time, the microcosm/macrocosm dissolves in a reverse order until it reaches the primordial state of equilibrium of the three gunas in Prakriti. This is said to be the end of one "cosmic cycle." This process is repeated again and again for an infinite number of times. This is personified as the all-manifesting and all-devouring cosmic form of the Lord shown in plate 2.

TABLE I. EVOLUTION ACCORDING TO YOGA

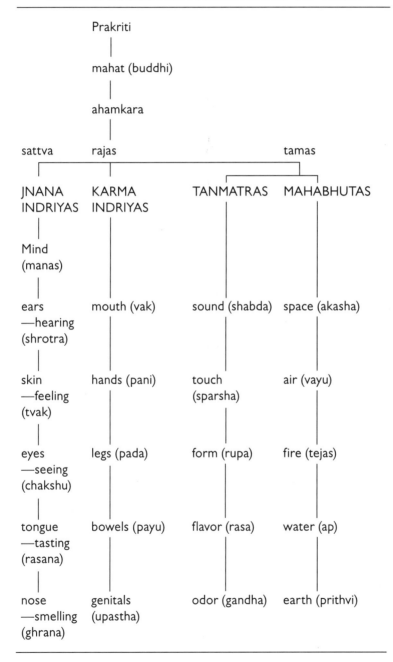

	Prakriti		
	mahat (buddhi)		
	ahamkara		
sattva	rajas		tamas
JNANA INDRIYAS	KARMA INDRIYAS	TANMATRAS	MAHABHUTAS
Mind (manas)			
ears —hearing (shrotra)	mouth (vak)	sound (shabda)	space (akasha)
skin —feeling (tvak)	hands (pani)	touch (sparsha)	air (vayu)
eyes —seeing (chakshu)	legs (pada)	form (rupa)	fire (tejas)
tongue —tasting (rasana)	bowels (payu)	flavor (rasa)	water (ap)
nose —smelling (ghrana)	genitals (upastha)	odor (gandha)	earth (prithvi)

Vital Energy

The second concept underlying the ancient system of the harmony of breath is that of the vital energy of vayu (air). The life of all living bodies depends upon the air that is breathed in and out. Without breathing life would not be possible. Similarly, the subtle body depends on the vital energy of prana, which circulates throughout the body and flows in and out along with the physical breath. Like the physical breath, prana energy also needs to be constantly replenished from the universal energy that pervades the cosmos.

As the normal rate of respiration in human beings is about fifteen breaths per minute, this adds up to a total of about 21,600 respirations every twenty-four hours. The vital energy (prana) that sustains the subtle body also flows in and out with the gross breath. As life depends on the process of breathing, and as some vital energy is lost during respiration, it is quite natural that if the rate of inhalation and exhalation is controlled and reduced, the vital energy can be preserved and life prolonged. Some yogis are said to have lived for many centuries or become immortal by carefully halting the flow of their vital energy.

The in and out flow of the vital energy along with the breath has observable effects on the human body. The claims made by yogis that they can stop their heartbeats and reduce the rate of respiration have been scientifically studied. Well-known experiments were conducted with Yogi Ramananda, who was sealed in an airtight metal box for up to ten hours. As he went into a trance, air samples measuring his body's oxygen uptake and heartbeat were monitored every half hour. These experiments showed dramatically that yogis were indeed capable of slowing normal body processes.[5] Yogis claim that if the flow of vital energy can be brought under conscious control, diseases can be prevented or cured, the course of human destiny altered, and a deep insight into the past and the future can be gained.

The Subtle Body

Within the subtle body are numerous channels or subtle pathways known as *nadis*, through which the vital energy of prana circulates all over the body. These are subtle and invisible vessels, and they have a psychic, not a physical, reality. These 72,000 subtle channels rise from the base of the spinal cord at the pelvic plexus (*muladhara chakra*) and spread throughout the body like veins through a leaf of the pipal tree (*Ficus religiosa*) (see plate 3).

There are twenty-four principal nadis: ten supply parts of the body above the navel, ten feed parts below the navel, and one pair of nadis branch to each side of the body. Ten out of the twenty-four principal channels are given special importance. Their names are: *ida, pingala, sushumna, gandhari, hastijihva, pusha, yashasvini, alambusha, kuhu,* and *shankhini.* These ten nadis that rise from the pelvic plexus terminate in special parts of the body. The ida terminates in the left nostril, the pingala in the right nostril, and the sushumna at the highest point of the cranium traditionally known as the *brahmarandhra* (aperture of immensity) and situated at the center of the dome of the skull. The gandhari ends in the left eye, the hastijihva in the right eye, the pusha in the right ear, the yashasvini in the left ear, the alambusha in the mouth, the kuhu in the genitals, and the shankhini in the anus.

Like the subtle nadis, there are ten currents of the vital energy of prana that circulate through the body. Five of these belong to the inner body: *prana, apana, samana, udana,* and *vyana.* They are collectively described as the *pancha pranas.* Prana circulates in the region of the heart, apana in the sphere of the anus, samana in the navel region, udana in the throat, and vyana pervades the whole body. In the evolutionary order, prana is related to the element fire and the sense of sight, apana to the element earth and the sense of smell, samana to the element water and the sense of taste, udana to the element air and the sense of touch, and vyana to the element space and the sense of hearing. According to the ancient tradition of the Prashnopanishad (III, 7), the vital energy of udana is the vehicle of the soul and is said to guide it from one body to another after death.

The pranas of the outer body are: *naga* for belching, vomiting, and giving rise to awareness; *kurma* for vision and opening and closing of the eyelids; *krikala* as the source of hunger and thirst, the flow of gastric juices, and for sneezing; *devadatta* for yawning; and *dhananjaya* for the distribution of nourishment to the subtle body. The last named vital energy is also said to pervade the entire body for a long time after death.

Ida, Pingala, and Sushumna

The three most important nadis of the subtle body are ida, pingala, and sushumna. Ida—frequently called the moon or Prakriti channel—is situated on the left and so rules all the nadis of the left half of the body. Pingala—called the sun channel and the symbol of the Purusha principle—rules the nadis on the right side of the body.

This left and right division of the subtle body and the nature of the psychic nadis has its parallels in modern scientific physiology of the brain. According to the most recent studies[6] the large and specialized cerebral cortex of the human brain is divided into two hemispheres, joined by a large bundle of fibers known as the corpus callosum. The left side of the body is controlled mainly by the right side of the cortex, and the right side of the body by the left cortex.

The structure and function of these two halves of the brain underlie the two modes of consciousness that coexist within each one of us. Although each hemisphere has the potential for many functions and both sides share and participate in many activities, in most normal persons the two hemispheres tend to specialize. The left hemisphere is predominantly involved in analytical and logical thinking, verbal skills, writing and speech, and complex mathematical calculations; the right hemisphere is concerned with synthesis, artistic and musical abilities, body image, recognition of faces, nonverbal (symbolic) ideas, creativity, and holistic thinking. Generally, right-left specialization is most prevalent in right-handed men but is slightly different in women and left-handers.

The third important nadi of the subtle body is the sushumna; it joins the center of the skull to the pelvic plexus and is known as the *meru danda*—the axis of the human body. Sushumna represents the perfect balance between the two polarities of right and left, sun and moon, Purusha and Prakriti, consciousness and energy.

Hidden inside the core of the sushumna nadi is an extra subtle channel called the *vajrani,* which runs the entire length of the sushumna. Within the vajrani is another subtle pathway known as the *chitrani* through which runs the shining Brahma nadi, the cause of yogic samadhi and enlightenment. This is how the famous text, the Shat Chakra Nirupana, describes these extra subtle pathways:

> She (Chitrani and the Brahma nadi) is beautiful like a chain of lightning and fine like a lotus fiber, and shines in the minds of sages. She is subtle; the awakener of pure knowledge; the embodiment of bliss and pure consciousness. The Brahma-dvara, entrance to the region of ambrosia, shines in her mouth (verse 3).[7]

Cleaning the Nadis

Just as the physical body needs to be cleaned and exercised to keep it in good health, the subtle body, and especially the channels, need to be cleaned frequently. The cleaning of the channels is called *nadi shodhana* and can be done both physically (*nirmanu*) and mentally (*samanu*). The physical methods include six yogic *kriyas* (actions) that need to be learned from a yogi guru. These kriyas are as follows:

1. *Kapalabhati*—stimulating the brain with abdominal and diaphragmatic breathing
2. *Neti*—cleaning the air passage with water, cotton strips, and milk
3. *Dhauti*—cleaning the intestinal tract

4. *Nauli*—isolation and rolling manipulation of the rectus abdominus muscles

5. *Trataka*—gazing at a fixed, generally bright, object to clear the eye channels

6. *Bhastrika*—rapid breathing or hyperventilation

✤

MENTAL CLEANSING OF THE NADIS

The mental methods of cleaning the nadis are many. The most important and common method includes mantra, meditation, and pranayama (breath control).

1. Sit in padmasana or siddhasana (see fig. 1.1 on page 9). Keep the gaze fixed on the tip of the nose all the time and meditate on *yam*, the mantra of air, which should be visualized as smoky in color and set in a crescent.

2. Inhale through the left nostril repeating the mantra *yam* six times.

3. Retain the breath, repeating *yam* twenty-four times, and then exhale slowly repeating the same mantra twelve times.

4. After this, meditate on the fire mantra *ram,* which is red and set in a flaming triangle. Inhale through the right nostril and repeat *ram* six times.

5. Retain the breath, repeating *ram* twenty-four times, and then exhale with the mantra repeated twelve times.

This entire exercise can be done for about ten rounds at first, increasing it gradually to what is suggested by the guru.

The Chakras

Strung along the central nadi, sushumna, are six basic chakras (psychic centers) that can be discovered and seen only by certain acts of introspection or dhyana (see fig. 1.2 on page 30). The lowest chakra is at the base of the spine, roughly between the anus and the genitals. This is called the *muladhara* (basic support) chakra and is identified with the pelvic plexus. Its form is that of a four-petaled red lotus with a yellow square in the center. On the four petals are inscribed, in gold, the letters (*matrikas*) *va, sha* (palatal), *sha* (lingual), and *sa* (dental) of the Sanskrit alphabet. Within the central yellow square is an inverted triangle, the symbol of the *yoni* (female genitalia), inside which is set a *lingam* (phallus). Coiled around the opening of the lingam lies the dormant spiritual power called *kundalini* (coiled) energy, represented visually as a serpent.

The power called kundalini is another form of the cosmic energy of Prakriti that animates all life. Kundalini is also the power of all psychological drives and motivations and the foundation of all emotions. According to the Tantra texts (Tantras), kundalini is composed of the three potential qualities (gunas) of nature and the energy of will (*iccha*),

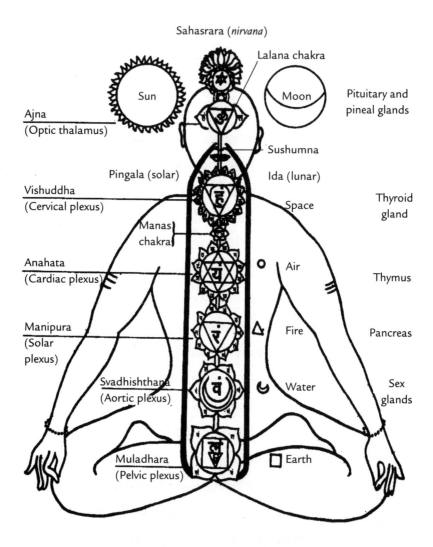

Sahasrara (*nirvana*)

Lalana chakra

Sun

Moon

Pituitary and
pineal glands

Ajna
(Optic thalamus)

Sushumna

Pingala (solar)

Ida (lunar)

Vishuddha
(Cervical plexus)

Space

Thyroid
gland

Manas
chakra

Anahata
(Cardiac plexus)

Air

Thymus

Manipura
(Solar
plexus)

Fire

Pancreas

Svadhishthana
(Aortic plexus)

Water

Sex
glands

Muladhara
(Pelvic plexus)

Earth

Fig. 1.2. The chakras of the subtle body

knowledge (*jnana*), and actions (kriyas). The famous Tara Rahasya Tantra describes the form of kundalini as "shining like ten million suns, cool like ten million moons, flashing like lightning in the sky, but also without form like the Immensity, Brahman" (IV, 24).

The muladhara, which is near the end of the alimentary canal, represents our fundamental concern as animals with digestion and excretion.

Near the genitals lies the second subtle chakra known as the *svadhishthana* (seat of the self). This chakra is depicted as a vermilion lotus with six petals, each inscribed with one of the following Sanskrit letters: *ba, bha, ma, ya, ra,* and *la.* The central area of this lotus is silver white, inset with a small crescent.

The svadhishthana is identified with the aortic plexus and symbolizes our most important drive after food, that of sexual gratification and reproduction.

At the level of the navel is the *manipura* (jewel-city) chakra, delineated as a lotus with ten blue petals. Each petal is marked with one of these Sanskrit letters: *da, dha, na* (lingual), *ta, tha, da, dha, na* (dental), *pa,* and *pha.* At the center is a red triangle with its apex pointing upward. This chakra is the seat of the vital energy called samana and represents the solar plexus. The goddess associated with this chakra, Lakini, is shown in plate 4.

Besides being the seat of samana, the manipura is also the center for the energy of ego (ahamkara). People who rise above the two basic animal concerns of food and sex usually stop at the ego center. Politicians, actors, business tycoons, and even some popular gurus who acquire important places in public life and attract followers usually have their entire energy concentrated in this center.

The *anahata* (vibrationless) chakra or the cardiac plexus is in the region of the heart, and is the home of prana, one of the five inner body vital energies. This chakra has twelve red—sometimes green—petals on which the Sanskrit letters *ka, kha, ga, gha, na, cha, chha, ja, jha, na, ta,* and *tha* (lingual) are inscribed in gold. The center of the anahata chakra is adorned by a double triangle making up a six-pointed star. The upward facing triangle symbolizes the lingam, and the downward pointing triangle stands for the yoni. Just above the anahata is a minor chakra called the *manas* chakra where the mind resides.

The anahata is the first center where the basic physical energy of the human being changes into spiritual energy. This is the center of compassion (*karuna*) and love (*prema*) and blooms only after a person is mature enough to rise above the usual physical and ego drives. The anahata is often called the home of the soul (*atman*). According to some yogic traditions, the higher mind, that is, the mind that is not entirely engrossed in physical matters, resides near and above this center of compassion. This chakra is called anahata because only when the energy becomes concentrated here does one hear the inner, nonvibratory (anahata) sound. This anahata sound is the aim of the *soham sadhana* described in chapter 4.

The *vishuddha* (pure) chakra is at the throat and is identified as the cervical plexus. This chakra can be visualized as a smoky purple lotus with sixteen petals, each marked with one of the vowels of the Sanskrit alphabet: *a, aa, i, ii, u, uu, ri, rii, lri, lrii, e, ai, o, au, am,* and *h.* In the center is a large blue arc of the moon. The vishuddha chakra is the seat of the inner-body vital energy called udana.

The vishuddha center is where the disciple gets the first glimpse of true samadhi (spiritual trance). Here all the basic psychological concerns are abandoned and the energy becomes purified. This is why the center is called vishuddha (pure).

Between the vishuddha and the higher *ajna* is a secret chakra called the *lalana* (female energy or the tongue). It is also known as the *talu* chakra because it is said to be situated at the base of the palate (talu) region just behind the uvula. Meditation on and visualization of this chakra is a secret to be learned from a guru. Some ancient tantrik texts say that the rising kundalini energy should be made to pass through the lalana center on its way to the ajna chakra. This can be accomplished with the help of the *hamsa* mantra (see chapter 4).

As it is a secret chakra, the description of the lalana differs from one text to another. According to the Saubhagya Lakshmi Upanishad (III, 6) the lalana chakra has twelve bright red petals. Other texts, however, say that the lalana has sixty-four silvery white petals and a bright red pericarp called the *ghantika* within which is the area (*bhumi*) of the moon's energy (*chandra kala*) from which sweet nectar oozes. It is said that when the disciple reaches the lalana chakra a sweet nectar starts dripping on the tongue. The lalana center is spiritually very important because it lies at the threshold of enlightenment and gives the *sadhaka* (practitioner) a glimpse of the great void (*maha shunya*).

The sixty-four petals of the lalana chakra are the homes of the powerful sixty-four (*chatuh shashti*) yoginis whose worship is said to grant the eight superhuman powers known as *siddhis*. Many gurus who exhibit magical abilities are usually stuck at this center and cannot rise above it.

Between the eyebrows, at the site of the third eye of Shiva (see plate 5), is the *ajna* (knowledge) chakra in the form of a white lotus with only two petals. On one petal is inscribed the letter *ha* and on the other the letter *ksha*. In the center of the lotus is a white, inverted triangle (yoni) within which is the lingam called the "other" (*itara*). The lingam in the ajna chakra is called itara in order to distinguish it from the lingam in the lowest chakra, the muladhara. The lingam in the muladhara represents animal drives, while the itara lingam in the ajna stands for animal energy transformed into spiritual power.

The itara lingam and the downward pointing white triangle symbolize the union of polarities, of Shiva (male) and Parvati (female), or of consciousness (Purusha) and energy (Prakriti), in the form of the divine hermaphrodite Ardhanarishvara (see plate 6).

A little beyond the ajna chakra is the *manas* (mind) center, which lies within chitrani nadi that runs through the sushumna channel. According to some traditions, the manas chakra is said to occupy the dot (*bindu*) that is part of the Omkara (the Sanskrit inscription of OM) at the center of the ajna. The visual form of the manas chakra has six petals, one each for the five senses—smell (earth), taste (water), form (fire), touch (air), and sound (space)—and the sixth one for sleep. The colors of the petals are related to the colors of the five elements—yellow (earth), white (water), red (fire), grey (air), white (space), and black for sleep. Manas chakra is the seat of consciousness where all modifications of the mind are absorbed.

Beyond the manas chakra is the *sahasrara padma*

(thousand-petaled lotus) whose petals encircle the dome of the skull and go beyond it into the cosmos. This is the center of bliss, the experience of utter joy. On the petals of this cosmic lotus are written all the possible sounds (50 x 20) of the Sanskrit language. In the center of this thousand-petaled lotus sit Shiva and Parvati in union. This is the end of the kundalini path. (See plate 7 for a depiction of the three highest chakras and their presiding deities.)

The symbol of Shiva and Parvati in union is a significant one. In the ajna center the polarities appear as a hermaphrodite, neither a complete male nor a complete female. This means that at the time of the opening of the eye of wisdom in the ajna center, sexuality is entirely transformed into spiritual energy. To represent this concept, Shiva and Parvati in the ajna chakra have no definite sexual nature. But beyond the ajna chakra, when the final bliss comes with the opening of the thousand-petaled lotus, sexuality may reestablish itself, shown by Shiva and Parvati having regained their individual sexuality and coming together in sexual union.

Bandhas and Mudras

The kundalini power that lies dormant at the base of the spine can be awakened by yogic techniques of neuromuscular locks (*bandhas*). Once awakened, the kundalini rises through the six chakras of the subtle body and ends in the sahasrara to give absolute bliss to the spiritual aspirant.

A word of warning: the bandhas and mudras are to be performed only under the practical instructions of an accomplished yogi-guru. If done without proper guidance, they can be very dangerous. The descriptions given here simply provide a general idea.

The first neuromuscular lock is called the *uddiyana* (flying-up) bandha and is performed by first exhaling all the air from the lungs through the mouth. Then, the chest is expanded and the abdominal muscles are sucked in so that they almost touch the backbone (detailed instructions on the performance of this bandha are given in chapter 3). The second lock is the *jalandhara* (glottis) bandha. It is performed by inhaling first through the nose and then contracting the throat so as to stop the air from going further. The chin is pressed firmly on the chest at the jugular notch. The third lock is called the *mula* (anus) bandha. It is done with the left heel against the perineum and the right heel above the genital region and the anus contracted.

There are many postures (*mudras*) that produce somatic electrochemical forces that can be used to awaken the kundalini energy. These are difficult to learn from a book and therefore not described here, with the exception of one as a sample. The *ashvini* (horse-like) mudra is performed by retaining the breath and rhythmically contracting the anal sphincter muscles about ten to thirteen times, each rhythm lasting about ten seconds. This mudra is said to quickly awaken the kundalini.

The Lokas

If the human body is compared to the cosmic body of Lord Shiva, who pervades the entire universe of planets, stars, space, and galaxies, the chakras described above can be called levels of existence or worlds (*lokas*).

The first is the world of material bodies and physical forces governed by natural laws. This is called the *jada loka* and represents the muladhara chakra. The second is the realm of life and vital energies, which are under the rule of biological laws. This is the *prana loka,* comparable to the svadhishthana center. The third world is called the *manas loka,* the world of mental forces that transcends matter and life, governed by subtle mental laws. This is the manipura chakra. The fourth world is the realm of the intellect, the *buddhi loka.* This realm rules the mind and corresponds to the anahata center. The fifth world is even higher and more subtle than the intellect. This is known as the realm of consciousness and is called the *dharma loka.* This world is comparable to the fifth center, vishuddha. In the cosmic body, the dharma loka governs the process of subtle evolution. Beyond the dharma loka is the world of pure divine beauty.

This is known as the *rasa loka* and it is where Shiva becomes his own beloved Parvati. The ajna chakra of wisdom corresponds to this world. The highest world is the *ananda loka* of pure bliss. The thousand-petaled lotus also represents this state of pure bliss in the human body. A symbolic depiction of the chakras of the cosmic body can be seen in plate 8.

Chapter Two

SVARODAYA
SHASTRA

*I*n the description of the physiology of the subtle body two important channels were mentioned: the ida and the pingala. The ida ends in the left nostril and pingala in the right nostril. The vital energy that flows through these two nadis flows in and out through the respective nostrils along with the physical breath. Just as we do not generally breathe equally through both nostrils simultaneously, only one of the two nadis is fully open at any given time. Yogis have observed that the vital breath flows through each nostril for approximately two and a half *ghatikas;* as one ghatika is equal to about twenty-four minutes, the change happens roughly once an hour.

The vital breath flowing through the right nostril is known as the sun (*surya*) svara, which is warm and excitable. The vital breath in the left nostril is called the moon (*chandra*) svara and is always cool and peaceful. When the vital breath changes from one nostril to the other, the action is known as the *svara samkranti.* Occasionally, when both the nostrils open up, this rare phenomenon is the *vishuvat kala,* or equal time. Texts refer to the open nostril as *purna* (full) and the closed nostril as *rikta* (empty) and the outgoing breath as *nirguna* (without attributes) and the incoming breath as *saguna* (with attributes).

Many great yogis of the past have carefully observed the relationship between the various events that happen in nature, the human physical and psychological states, and the changes of the vital breath from one nostril to the other. They have recorded this knowledge in several texts that have been kept diligently hidden and revealed only rarely to serious students of Yoga and astrology. Yogis claim that a master of the svarodaya shastra can predict the future course of events on Earth, can prevent and cure diseases, both physical and mental, and can influence the work of nature in matters such as the determination of the sex of an unborn child. Not all these methods are known, and the available texts mention only a few. Many are said to have been lost because of the break in the ancient *guru-shishya* (teacher-disciple) tradition. The rest have to be learned from a master guru.

The Basic Rules for the Movement of the Vital Breath

The movement of the vital breath is addressed by a number of different theories. The first states that during the bright half (*shukla paksha*) of the lunar month, the first, second, third, seventh, eighth, ninth, thirteenth, fourteenth, and fifteenth (full moon) days should begin with the vital breath in the moon—left—nostril. The moon is the lord of the left nadi and the bright half of the month, so the theory is that its power and influence is greatest during this period. Therefore the left breath is most auspicious at the beginning (1, 2, 3), middle (7, 8, 9) and end (13, 14, 15) of the bright lunar half. During the remaining six days (4, 5, 6 and 10, 11, 12) the power of the moon is low and so the days should start with the vital breath flowing through the right, solar nostril.

This process is reversed in the dark half (*krishna paksha*) of the lunar month when the sun is powerful and influential at the beginning, middle, and end of the period. Any long-term change from this basic pattern, if not accompanied by other compensating good and auspicious factors, may signify a period of trouble and many setbacks. It is advisable not to start any new important venture during such a period.

According to another theory, given in one text of the svarodaya shastra, the breath should be in the left nostril at sunrise on odd days of the bright half of the lunar month, and in the right nostril on even days. This is reversed during the dark half of the month.

An oral tradition states that the breath should change from one nostril to the other every three days starting with the left nostril on the first day of the bright half of the lunar month.

Traditionally, lunar *panchangas* (five limbs of time) were

regarded as essential to determine the correct day. The five limbs are: the solar day (day of the week), the lunar day, the *nakshatra* (star constellations of Indian astrology), the conjunction of planets, and halves of lunar days. Today, lunar months are not generally used, so a more simple and direct method is also used, in which the day of the week is given more importance than the lunar day.

As the breath flowing through the left nostril is considered cooler than the vital breath of the right nostril, days associated with the moon (*chandra* or *soma*) should begin with the left nostril open: Monday (Somavara = day of the moon), Wednesday (Budhavara = day of Mercury), Thursday (Guruvara = day of Jupiter), and Friday (Shukravara = day of Venus). The astrological reason for this association is that the moon and Mercury are friends, while the moon, Jupiter, and Venus are neutrals.

The right nostril represents the sun and so the vital breath from this channel is warm. Therefore, it should flow from the right nostril on Sunday (Ravivara = day of the sun), Tuesday (Mangalavara = day of Mars), and Saturday (Shanivara = day of Saturn). Astrologically Sun and Mars are friends, and even though Sun and Saturn are enemies, according to Indian mythology Saturn (Shani) is the son of the sun (Ravi-putra).

These various theories regarding the movement of the vital breath are summarized in the following table.

TABLE 2. METHODS OF DETERMINING THE AUSPICIOUS INITIAL BREATH FOR A GIVEN DAY

Left (moon nadi)	Right (sun nadi)
First theory	
bright half	
1, 2, 3, 7, 8, 9, 13, 14, 15	4, 5, 6, 10, 11, 12
dark half	
4, 5, 6, 10, 11, 12	1, 2, 3, 7, 8, 9, 13, 14, 15 (new moon)
Second theory	
bright half	
odd days—1, 3, 5, and so on	even days—2, 4, 6, and so on
dark half	
even days	odd days
Third theory—change every third day	
Fourth theory (day of the week theory)	
Monday, Wednesday, Thursday, Friday	Sunday, Tuesday, Saturday

BLOCKING THE VITAL BREATH IN ONE NOSTRIL

In order to avoid the misfortunes that can be triggered by beginning a given day with the breath in the wrong nostril, it may be necessary to block the flow of vital breath through one of the two nostrils, which will cause the dominance to switch. This can be done in four very simple ways.

Alternate Nostril Breathing

Breathe in deeply through the open nostril, and then breathe out through the closed nostril. Do this about ten or twenty times and the flow of vital breath will change from one nostril to the other.

Lying on Your Side

Lie on a flat, hard bed on your side. You should lie on the side corresponding to the closed nostril, and within a few minutes it will open up.

Blocking with Cotton Wool

The third method will be described more fully later, but in short, it involves the blocking of the open nostril with a small wad of cotton wool.

Using the Yoga Danda

The fourth method involves the use of the yoga danda. Place the yoga danda under the armpit on the side of the open nostril and lean over and press it between the chest and the arm. Maintain this position for about 15 minutes and the breath will change to the nostril on the side opposite to the yoga danda.

The first two methods of changing the flow of the vital breath can be used when only one or two changes in a day are required. But if the vital breath has to be kept confined to only one nostril for a long time, the third and fourth methods are more practical. There is a subtle fifth method of changing the vital breath, but this is based on deep meditation and is difficult to understand without a guru.

The Five Elements of the Vital Breath

As already mentioned, the vital breath flows through each nostril for about an hour. But within this hour, the quality, intensity, and power of the vital breath does not remain the same throughout. There are at least five subtle, important, and noticeable changes that the vital breath undergoes. These changes are traditionally correlated to the five elements (*tattvas*): earth (prithvi), water (ap), fire (tejas), air (vayu), and space (akasha). These are of course not the material elements of everyday life, but states of subtle matter that affect the physical, emotional, and psychic processes of the human body.

There are many outer (physical) and inner (meditative) ways of identifying the five elements of the vital breath. Each element has many and varied characteristics that help in their identification, including the nature of the breath, time of flow, type of breath, manner of flow, length of flow, geometrical shape, color, taste, experience of seed (*bija*) mantra, and physical manifestation.

The Nature and Time of Flow of the Breath Elements

In a given hour the breath changes to manifest the characteristics of each of the elements.

- The breath of the earth element is slow, slightly warm, makes a deep sound, and has a central flow that seems to stem from the chin. The breath lasts for about 20 minutes.
- The breath of the water element flows very fast, makes a very loud sound, is cold to the touch, and lasts for about 16 minutes.
- The fire element breath is very hot and lasts for 12 minutes.

- The air element breath can be either hot or cold and lasts for 8 minutes.
- The breath of the space element has the combined characteristics of the other elements and lasts for only 4 minutes.

After every 60 minutes the flow of vital breath moves over to the next nostril where the above process is repeated.

A different tradition based on another text gives this short guide to the identification of the breath element: in the 60-minute period of the vital breath flowing from any one nostril, the first 10 minutes are of the space element, then 14 minutes of the earth element, 12 minutes of the water element, 12 minutes of the air element, and the last 12 minutes of the fire element.

The Length of Flow

The length of flow of the different elements is measured in finger-breadths, or *angulas.*

- Earth is 12 angulas
- Water is 16 angulas
- Fire is 4 angulas
- Air is 8 angulas
- Space is 20 angulas

❦

DETERMINING THE LENGTH OF THE BREATH
TO IDENTIFY THE ELEMENT

The method of determining the length of the breath is as follows.

1. Lay very well separated cotton wool or very fine sand on a flat surface and hold it near the open nostril.

2. Exhale through that nostril at normal rate and carefully note where the maximum movement of the cotton wool or sand takes place.

3. The distance of the site of maximum movement from the nostril is the length of the breath, which will indicate which breath element is active.

The Direction of Flow of the Breath Elements

When the vital breath flows out of the open nostril, its direction is determined by the element that is active at the time. Breath of the earth element flows from the center of the nostril, water element flows downward, while the flow of the fire element is upward. Air element breath flows from the side of the nostril and the space element flows with equal force all over.

Other Characteristics of the Breath Elements

Each breath element has a characteristic geometric shape, color, and taste.

- **Earth:** square, yellow or golden, sweet
- **Water:** crescent, white, astringent
- **Fire:** triangle, red, pungent
- **Air:** circle, green, sour
- **Space:** a point (bindu), multicolored, bitter

DETERMINING THE BREATH ELEMENT
BY OBSERVATION

Outer Method

The outer method of determining the current breath element is to hold a small, clean mirror or a piece of clean glass near the open nostril and then breathe out at a normal rate. The geometric shape that the condensation takes—square, crescent, triangle, circle, or dots—indicates the breath element.

Inner Method

The inner method of determining the current breath element is as follows.

1. Find a quiet, clean place, far away from human habitation and worldly distractions.

2. Sit either in the siddhasana or the padmasana (as shown in fig. 1.1 on page 9).

3. Having taken up either of the two asanas, perform the *shanmukhi* (six-faced) mudra (fig. 2.1). This mudra is done by gently pressing and shutting the ears with the thumbs, the eyes with the index fingers, the nose with the middle fingers, the lips with the ring fingers, and letting the pinkie fingers rest on the chin. At first concentrate on your chosen deity and then slowly try to clear your mind of all disturbing thoughts.

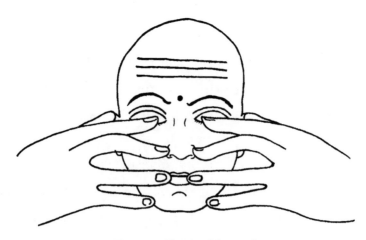

Fig. 2.1. Shanmukhi mudra

After the mind has become concentrated, if you see a yellow or golden square and your mouth becomes filled with a sweet taste, this is the flow of the earth element. If a white crescent appears along with an astringent taste in the mouth, this is the water element. The appearance of a red triangle and a pungent taste on the tongue indicates the flow of the fire element. The air element will materialize as a green circle and a sour taste in the mouth. The space element will become visible as multicolored dots. At the same time the mouth will fill up with a bitter taste.

The Natural Order of the Breath Elements

According to some svarodaya texts, the natural order of the breath elements can be correlated to the days of the week, so that at sunrise on Sunday, the day should begin with the breath in the earth element, Monday in the water element, Tuesday in the fire element, Wednesday in the earth element again, Thursday in the air element, Friday in the fire element, and Saturday in the space element.

Seed (Bija) Mantras of the Vital Breath Elements

Each element is associated with a seed or bija mantra: earth—*lam;* water—*vam;* fire—*ram;* air—*yam;* space— *ham.* To experience the reality of the various elements of the vital breath through their bija mantras, a special form of meditation is recommended, which is based on the association of the elements and the chakras.

❦

EXPERIENCING THE REALITY OF THE
BREATH ELEMENTS

1. After the first quarter of the night has passed, find a pure, clean secluded place. Sit on a grass mat in the *vajrasana* (thunderbolt) posture. This posture is formed by kneeling on the ground with the heels under the buttocks (fig. 2.2).

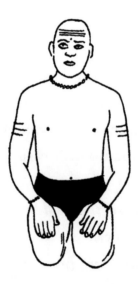

Fig. 2.2. The thunderbolt posture—vajrasana

2. Then meditate, letting your vital breaths, mental functions, and the kundalini power identify with the elements at the chakras one by one, moving from the gross to the most subtle, as meditation and absorption deepen. This is the process of laya yoga, by which the individual identity is dissolved into the supreme consciousness.

3. At first you will experience reality as solid matter (earth) through the visualization of the seed mantra *lam* in the muladhara center.

4. Then, with the appearance of *vam,* the bija mantra of the svadhishthana chakra, you will move upward, and know reality in the fluid state (water).

5. In the seed mantra *ram* lies the manipura chakra where reality is consumed by fire and all sense of time is transcended.

6. When the bija *yam* appears before the mind's eye, you will penetrate the cosmic air and hear the sound produced without vibrations (anahata).

7. Beyond this is the realm of the vishuddha chakra and the seed mantra *ham.* This level of realization is beyond all earthly wisdom, and cannot be described by words. It is as vast as space.

8. When your consciousness reaches the level of the ajna chakra between the eyebrows, you have reached the state of formless contemplation (*asamprajnata samadhi*).

Here the bija mantra is the cosmic word of power, OM.

9. Beyond the ajna chakra is the awareness of infinity in the sahasrara chakra.

The Physical Manifestations of the Five Elements

The physical manifestations of the five elements in the human body are as follows:

Earth: bones, flesh, skin, veins, and hair

Water: semen, blood, marrow, urine, and saliva

Fire: hunger, thirst, sleep, lust, and sloth

Air: running, walking, bending, contracting, and expanding

Space: anger, energy, shame, fear, and lust

It goes without saying that control over the vital breaths of the five elements gives full control over their corresponding physical manifestations.

The breath of the five elements should flow in the regular manner already explained. Any long term irregularity can cause diseases such as jaundice and asthma. The table on the next page gives the diseases that can be caused by the uneven flow of the elements of the vital breath:

TABLE 3. DISEASES CAUSED BY UNEVEN ELEMENT
FLOW IN THE VITAL BREATH

Element	Quality	Organ of perception	Organ of action	Disease
Earth	Smell	Nose	Anus	Jaundice
Water	Taste	Tongue	Penis	Hallucination
Fire	Form	Eyes	Feet	Swellings
Air	Touch	Skin	Hands	Asthma
Space	Sound	Ears	Mouth	—

In the human body the water element rules the feet, earth element the knees, air the groins, fire the chest and shoulders, and space the head.

The breath elements also have a very profound effect upon the mind. When the earth element is rising, there is calmness and peace that cannot be disturbed by the most serious problems. With the rising of the water element breath, the mind becomes filled with joy and compassion and there is a tremendous inner need to help others. Breath of the fire element brings with it anger, mental turmoil, violence, pride, and terror. When the breath of the air element is rising the mind becomes disturbed and restless like

TABLE 4. QUALITIES ASSOCIATED WITH THE FIVE VITAL BREATH ELEMENTS

Element	Place in the Body	Shape	Quality	Color	Taste	Mantra	Length	Time	Nature	Direction	Effect
Earth	anus (muladhara chakra)	square	smell	yellow	sweet	*lam*	12 angulas	20 minutes	equitable	east	beneficial after a long time
Water	genitals (svadhishthana chakra)	crescent	taste	white	astringent	*vam*	16 angulas	16 minutes	peaceful	west	quick benefit
Fire	navel (manipura chakra)	triangle	form	red	pungent	*ram*	4 angulas	12 minutes	pain and friction	south	no effect
Air	heart (anahata chakra)	circle	touch	smoky	sour	*yam*	8 angulas	8 minutes	excitable	north	small benefit
Space	throat (vishuddha chakra)	bindu	sound	many-colored	bitter	*ham*	20 angulas	4 minutes	confusion	center	none

the wind. Space element breath has a calming effect on the mind. There arises an inner need to meditate and this is the best time for spiritual discipline.

Astrology and Svara

According to the Tantras, the distinction between the breath from the left and right nostrils is due to the movements of the celestial bodies. Indian astrology observes the movement of the moon through a different set of constellations than those of the Western zodiac. These constellations, or "asterisms," are called *nakshatras* in Sanskrit, and are identified by their prominent stars. There are 28 nakshatras, one for each day of the lunar cycle; they are also referred to as the "lunar mansions." Astrologers say that just as the breath elements influence human behavior and destiny, so do the nakshatras, or asterisms. According to the Shiva Svarodaya Shastra, "As the moon moves through the signs of the zodiac, so the breath moves from the moon (left) nostril to the sun (right) nostril." An individual's zodiac sign determines which breath is beneficial on which day.

A correlation has been established between the asterisms and the five elements of the vital breath. In the list below each element is shown with its corresponding (numbered) nakshatras and their prominent stars.

Earth: (1) Dhanishtha (Alpha, Beta, Gamma, and Delta Delphinis), (2) Rohini (Aldebaran), (3) Jyeshtha (Alpha, Sigma, and Tau Scorpionis), (4) Anuradha (Beta, Delta, and Pi Scorpionis), (5) Shravana (Alpha, Beta, and Gamma Aquilae), (6) Abhijit (Alpha, Epsilon, and Zeta Lyrae), and (7) Uttarashadha (Zeta and Sigma Sagittarii).

Water: (8) Purvashadha (Delta and Epsilon Sagittarii), (9) Ashlesha (Delta, Epsilon, Eta, Rho, and Sigma Hydrae), (10) Mula (Epsilon, Zeta, Eta, Theta, Iota, Kappa, Lambda, Mu, and Upsilon Scorpionis), (11) Ardra (Alpha Orionis), (12) Revati (Zeta Piscium and so on), (13) Uttarabhadrapada (Gamma Pegasi and Alpha Andromedae), and (14) Shatabhisha (Gamma Aquarii).

Fire: (15) Bharani (35, 39, and 41 Arietis), (16) Krittika (Pleiades), (17) Pushya (Gamma, Delta, and Theta Cancri), (18) Magha (Alpha, Gamma, Epsilon, Zeta, Eta, and Mu Leonis), (19) Purvaphalguni (Delta and Theta Leonis), (20) Purvabhadrapada (Alpha and Beta Pegasi), and (21) Svati (Arcturus).

Air: (22) Vishakha (Alpha, Beta, Gamma, and Iota Librae), (23) Uttaraphalguni (Beta and 93 Leonis), (24) Hasta (Alpha, Beta, Gamma, Delta, and Epsilon Corvi), (25) Chitra (Spica and Alpha Virginis), (26)

Punarvasu (Alpha and Beta Geminorum), (27) Ashvini (Beta and Gamma Ariatis), and (28) Mrigashira (Lambda, Phi 1, and Phi 2 Orionis).

Space has no corresponding asterism.

According to astrologers there is also a relationship between the planets, the signs of the zodiac, and the breath elements. On the left (ida) channel, the earth element is influenced by Mercury, water by the moon, fire by Venus, and air by Jupiter. On the right (pingala) nadi, earth is under the rule of the sun, water under Saturn, fire under Mars, and air under the ascending node of the moon (rahu). On the central channel (sushumna), earth relates to Mercury, water to the moon and Venus, fire to the sun and Mars, air to the ascending node of the moon and Saturn, and space to Jupiter.

The twelve signs of the Western zodiac and the breath elements also influence each other; their relationship is as follows: earth—Taurus, Virgo, and Capricorn; water—Cancer, Scorpio, and Pisces; air—Gemini, Libra, and Aquarius; and fire—Aries, Leo, and Sagittarius. Space has no influence on the signs of the zodiac.

At this point, it would be useful to summarize all the relationships and associations of the three main nadis of the subtle body.

TABLE 5. SUMMARY OF RELATIONSHIPS IN
THE THREE MAIN NADIS

	Right	Left	Central
Nadi	pingala	ida	sushumna
Planet	Sun	Moon	Rahu (ascending node of the moon)
Nature	excitable	calm	mixed
Gender	male	female	neutral
Deity	Shiva	Shakti	Ardhanarishvara
Color	black	white	gray
Time	day	night	twilight
Element	fire and air	water and earth	space
Sign	unstable	stable	both
Day	Sunday, Tuesday, Saturday	Monday, Wednesday, Thursday, and Friday	Wednesday and Thursday
Lunar half	dark	bright	—
Lunar day (*tithi*)	dark: 1, 2, 3, 7, 8, 9, 13, 14, 15 (new moon); bright: 4, 5, 6, 10, 11, 12	bright 1, 2, 3, 7, 8, 9, 13, 14, 15 (full moon); dark: 4, 5, 6, 10, 11, 12	—

	Right	Left	Central
Lunar month	Vaishakha, Shravana, Karttika, and Magha	Jyeshtha, Bhadrapada, Margashirsha, and Phalguna	Ashadha, Ashwina, Pausha, and Chaitra
Passage (samkranti)	Aries, Gemini, Leo, Libra, Aquarius, and Sagittarius	Taurus, Cancer, Virgo, Scorpio, Capricorn, and Pisces	—
Sign of the zodiac	Aries, Cancer, Libra, and Capricorn	Taurus, Leo, Scorpio, and Aquarius	Gemini, Virgo, Sagittarius, and Pisces
Lunar asterisms	Ashvini, Bharani, Krittika, Utt. Shadha, Abhijit, Shravana, Dhanishtha, Shatabhisha, Revati, Pur. Bhadrapada, and Rohini	Ashlesha, Magha, Pur. Phalguni, Utt. Phalguni, Hasta, Chitra, Svati, Vishakha, Anuradha, Mula, Pur. Shadha, and Jyeshtha	Mrigashira, Ardra, Punarvasu, and Pushya
Direction	east and north	west and south	angle
Number	odd	even	zero

Chapter Three

SVARODAYA SHASTRA AND HUMAN DESTINY

*T*he subtle channels, chakras, vital breaths, and their functions in the subtle human body have all been explained. Now let us consider some of the effects of these subtle forces on human destiny, and the laws that give us the knowledge of these forces.

In the various activities we undertake, we find that no matter how hard we try we are not always rewarded with success. This is because—in addition to the many physical forces at work—there are hidden forces that influence our behavior. These forces generally remain unknown, though their effects are just as potent as those of the physical forces. But the subtle, hidden forces are not always beyond discovery. Many people in the past have been able to acquire the occult knowledge of svarodaya, and use their understanding of nadis, vital breaths, and subtle chakras for their benefit. And most of these people are not great yogis, but ordinary people like you and me. With devotion, faith, and serious study, the wisdom of svarodaya shastra can be learned and mastered by any sincere and virtuous person.

No intelligent person can fail to notice that the moods of human beings change very frequently. Sometimes we are happy and cheerful, while at other times we feel angry and depressed. Most people feel that these changing moods depend on outside stimuli only. This is not true. The flow of vital breath and its five elements have a strong influence on our temperament. Otherwise, how could sudden periods of depression followed by equally sudden periods of cheerfulness without any apparent reason be explained? So it stands to reason that if we can understand and control the movements of the vital breath, we can command and modify our moods, and indirectly influence our environment. The occult wisdom of svarodaya helps in doing just that.

The first general rule of svarodaya is that all auspicious activities aimed at obtaining permanent and stable effects should be undertaken when the vital breath is flowing through the left (moon) channel. Care should be taken to start the propitious acts within the first 90 *palas* (36 minutes) of the initiation of the flow of the vital breath in the left nostril. This is because the breath elements of earth and water—which flow in the first 20 and 16 minutes, respectively—are considered to be very beneficial, while the fire, air, and space elements—which follow—are said to be harmful.

Below is a short list of activities that can be initiated during the breath flow of the earth and water elements in the left channel.

- Making new jewelry, clothes, and icons
- Leaving home to go on a long journey, either toward the south or the west

- Entering a hermitage or a monastery
- Visiting a king, minister, or other state dignitary
- Beginning the construction of artificial lakes, dams, reservoirs, and ornamental gardens
- Erecting large public monuments, commemorative pillars, statues of kings, and important public figures
- Making and entering new houses
- Going on a pilgrimage
- Giving donations and performing other charitable acts
- Celebrating weddings and domestic rites meant to secure peace and good health
- Administering special tonics and herbal preparations to promote quick recovery from an illness
- Meeting friends, business partners, and employers
- Buying reserve stores of food grains
- Commencing first agricultural operations of the season
- Purchasing domestic animals
- Studying Yoga
- Casting spells and performing magical rituals to cure diseases and to secure good harvests

All the activities listed above bring especially favorable results if done on Wednesdays, Thursdays, or Fridays.

The right (sun) channel dominates evil, cruel, and difficult-to-accomplish acts. So, for best results, undertake these activities at a time when the vital breath is flowing through the right nostril in either the earth or water element.

A short list of acts one should engage in during the flow of the sun channel is given below:

- Learning and teaching magical arts
- Sexual intercourse with prostitutes
- Sailing in a new ship
- Making and drinking strong, fermented drinks
- Acquiring physical and psychic powers through the performance of magical charms and unorthodox rites that involve animal sacrifices
- Casting spells to confuse the enemy's mind; making *yantras* (mystical diagrams); and magically gaining control over vampires and zombies (*vetalas*), eaters of raw flesh (*pishachas*), ghosts (*pretas*), and wandering souls (*bhutas*)
- Climbing mountains and entering fortified cities
- Making and cutting bricks and fashioning building stones
- Cutting precious stones
- Plastering and decorating a new house
- Engaging in sword fights and duels

- Starting the study of difficult arts and sciences
- Establishing mental control over prostitutes and young virgins
- Eating very rich and difficult-to-digest food

Tuesdays, Saturdays, and Sundays are especially favorable for all the above tasks.

When the flow of the vital breath rapidly fluctuates from one nostril to the other, this denotes the flow of the central (sushumna) channel. This channel is like fire, and is said to burn all worldly pursuits. Therefore, when the vital breath flows through this nadi, suspend all secular occupations. Do not even curse or bless anyone. Just sit in a quiet, clean place and meditate on your chosen deity or on the formless, transcendental Reality. It is said in the ancient svarodaya texts that even rituals and pilgrimages are useless during the flow of the sushumna. This channel brings either death or spiritual bliss.

There is no need to take the word death here too literally. It is likely that the death referred to in the svarodaya texts is the end of the ego and not the death of the physical body. According to the Tantras, death of the "ego" is always considered to be the real death. Once the sense of "I-ness"—the sense that I am different from the cosmos— has gone, physical life or death loses its meaning. Death is no longer looked upon as annihilation, but as change from one level of consciousness to another.

Svarodaya and Sexual Relationships

The basic principles of vital breath that are described in the svarodaya Tantras apply equally to men and women. But it is necessary to remember that the solar channel symbolizes the male, and the lunar channel the female. Consequently, the power of the breath for a man is highest in the sun channel and for the woman in the moon channel. Naturally the moon channel of the female is attracted by the sun channel of the male, and vice versa. So if a man desires to completely enjoy a woman, he should approach her while his breath is in the right nostril and the woman's breath is in the left nostril. This is the best time for both of them to unite in sexual intercourse. In such a union they will get blissful satisfaction. In fact, if a married couple or two lovers observe this rule whenever they unite in sexual intercourse, their love will prosper like that of the mythical Rati (Psyche) and Kamadeva (Eros).

※

GAINING POWER OVER ANOTHER PERSON

If it is found necessary to influence a man or a woman whom you desire so that he or she will do as you wish, here is a practical method.

1. First determine the open nostril and the element of your breath.
2. Then take your first step toward the person, starting with the foot that coincides with the side of the open nostril.

If the above instructions are observed, the man or the woman of your desire and fancy will be within your power in a very short time.

There is a potent method for a man to gain control over a woman who rejects all his advances. This is a secret law, which the Tantras say should not be disclosed to a lecherous man. It is for the use of a good man whose love is deep and genuine.

※

A POTENT METHOD FOR A GOOD MAN
TO ATTRACT A WOMAN

1. Approach her when she is fast asleep.
2. If her breath is in the moon nostril, and your breath

happens to be in the sun nostril, then slowly uncover her "great lotus" (vulva) and blow your sun breath into it. Then leave her.

When she awakens she will develop a strong itch in her vagina, which will be relieved only by sexual intercourse with the man who filled her great lotus with his sun breath.

The Effects of Svarodaya on Unborn Children

Many women would like to predetermine the sex of their children. Failing this, they would be very happy if it were possible at least to have knowledge of the sex of the unborn child. Some of the occult methods based on the svarodaya system of predicting and in some cases predetermining the sex of an embryo are given below.

❦

PREDETERMINING THE SEX AND CHARACTER OF AN UNBORN CHILD

A woman is said to be fertile from the fourth to the sixteenth day after menstruation. She can become pregnant any time within this period. If the day she becomes pregnant happens to be the eighth, eleventh, thirteenth, fourteenth, or the fifteenth (either the full moon day or the day before the new moon) day of the lunar month, she will be blessed with a good looking and healthy male child.

The general rule for a woman who wants a male child is to have sexual intercourse within the fertile period and on one of the above-mentioned propitious days, whenever her left nostril and her husband's right nostril are open. The vital breath should be in the earth element.

The rule for a woman who desires a female child is to copulate within the fertile period and on the correct auspicious day when her husband's left nostril and her right nostril are flowing. The vital breath should be in the water element.

Below are enumerated some further details regarding the day on which a woman becomes pregnant, and its effect on the unborn child's character.

In an oral svarodaya tradition the effects of the breath elements on the unborn child are as follows:

1. If impregnation happens when the woman's breath is in the earth element, the child will become brave, adventurous, deep and thoughtful, charitable, religious, long living, and lucky. The child will have a very fair skin and a well-built and well-proportioned body.

TABLE 6. THE EFFECTS OF SVARODAYA
ON A MALE CHILD

Day after Menstruation	Qualities of the Child
Fourth	Thin and delicate boned
Sixth	Average health and life
Eighth	Lazy and pleasure-loving
Tenth	Clever
Twelfth	Clever and handsome
Fourteenth	Clever, handsome, and virtuous
Sixteenth	All imaginable good qualities

TABLE 7. THE EFFECTS OF SVARODAYA
ON A FEMALE CHILD

Day after Menstruation	Qualities of the Child
Fifth	Deformed and ugly
Seventh	Might be unhappy in old age
Ninth	Lazy and pleasure-loving
Eleventh	Easy morals
Thirteenth	Will marry a man of low caste
Fifteenth	Will become a queen

2. When the woman's breath is in the water element, the child will be good looking, fair, calm, friendly, very imaginative, pleasure-loving, and healthy.

3. If the mother's breath happens to be in the fire element, the child will be dark, excitable, proud, cruel, and coarse, but at the same time brave, muscular, and a good fighter who will make an excellent soldier. A child of the fire element can cause a difficult delivery.

4. If the mother becomes pregnant in the air element, she will deliver a child that is thin, pale, weak, lazy, and very unstable. Such a child will grow up to be talkative, untruthful, sly, a coward, and a mischief maker.

5. Pregnancies in the space element generally result in miscarriages, but if such a child does live, it will become a saint.

⁂

TO OVERCOME INFERTILITY

An infertile woman can bear a child if her husband copulates with her at a time when either her central channel has just opened, or her vital breath is flowing in the fire element of the sun nadi.

The rules mentioned above are very general. The subtle effects of the vital breaths and their elements on the unborn child can only be learned from a yogi. No number of books can teach the inner, hidden mysteries.

General Applications of Svarodaya to Influence Outcomes

The following three exercises outline techniques for influencing other people and for making the course of any given day auspicious.

❧

INFLUENCING A DIFFICULT PERSON

To bring about a favorable response from any person who is difficult to deal with, keep that person on the side of your open channel while you negotiate. This will make the person agreeable and responsive. This method works particularly well during business bargaining, court cases, and job interviews.

❧

INFLUENCING A PERSON FROM A DISTANCE

To influence a person at a great distance hold a shallow vessel full of clean water and face the direction in which the person to be influenced resides. Think of that person and try to suck some water through the open channel. If you are even slightly psychic this method will surely work.

❧

INFLUENCING THE COURSE OF THE DAY

To influence the course of the day and make it good and auspicious, do the following:

1. When you wake up in the morning, check which nostril is open.

2. Then rub your face with the hand on the side of the flowing channel.

3. As you step out of bed, touch the ground first with the foot on the side of the open nostril.

You will have good luck throughout the day.

Changes in the Natural Rhythm of the Vital Breath and Their Effects upon Health and Fortune

We now know what the normal pattern of breathing is, and how it changes from hour to hour and from day to day. If this pattern is disturbed either naturally or artificially, and remains altered for a long period, it usually denotes a change in health and fortune.

There are two ways in which the normal rhythm of breathing can be altered. If the day begins with the vital breath in the wrong nostril it is called the "day change." If the duration of flow through any one nostril either increases or decreases significantly, this is known as the "time change." The effects of these changes are:

Day Change

- If the day of the new moon commences with the vital breath in the right nostril instead of the left one, there are chances that the person concerned will, within a fortnight, suffer either from a mild fever or domestic quarrels or both.
- On the first day of the dark half of the lunar month, if the vital breath begins to flow in the left nostril at dawn, understand that there will be an attack of influenza or severe cold, as well as some financial loss.
- If any changed pattern of the flow of vital breath remains so for a whole lunar month there are strong chances of very serious misfortunes.
- If the disturbance in the flow of vital breath lasts for a fortnight, consider this as a forewarning of serious illness.

- If the changed pattern of breath passes away within three days, there is every reason to be grateful to God for having saved you from the coming of a serious disease. There might, however, be a slight headache and fever for a day or so as the result of the short change.

Time Change (Pleasant Effects)

- If the moon channel flows for 1 hour and 20 minutes, you may get a pleasant surprise.
- If the moon channel flows for 3 hours 10 minutes, there will be domestic peace.
- If the left nostril remains open continuously for 5 hours and 36 minutes, you will meet a long lost relative or friend.
- If the left nostril stays open for 24 hours, you will get a small fortune.
- If the flow of the vital breath through each nostril is prolonged by 30 minutes, and if the pattern remains unchanged for 48 hours, you will soon become very popular and famous.
- If anyone breathes through the moon nostril all day and the sun nostril all night, he will live to be 108.
- The unchanging flow of the moon channel for 4, 8, 12, or 20 days and nights, means a long and happy life.

Time Change (Unpleasant Effects)

- If the left channel flows nonstop for 4 hours, there will be frequent attacks of rheumatism or related disorders.
- If the left channel flows nonstop for 4 hours 48 minutes, there will be trouble from enemies.
- If the left channel flows nonstop for 1, 2, or 3 days, there will be physical suffering.
- If the left channel flows nonstop for 1 month, there will be heavy financial loss.
- If the right channel remains open without a break for 1 hour and 36 minutes, there is a possibility of stomach disorders such as ulcers and indigestion.
- If the right channel remains open without a break for 8 hours and 24 minutes, your friends are likely to turn against you.
- If the right channel remains open without a break for 24 hours, serious illness is likely.

Readjusting a Disturbed Breath Pattern

There is no need to panic or be depressed if the vital breath happens to flow in one of the negative manners described above. Diseases and unpleasant events can be either prevented or their intensity reduced by simply readjusting the disturbed breath pattern. To do this it is essential to block one nostril. This can be done by inserting a small wad of clean cotton wool wrapped in a little gauze into the nostril. It is, however, very important to remember not to smoke tobacco, shout, sing, or talk loudly, or to do strenuous physical work while the nostril is blocked.

General Rules Regarding Svarodaya and Good Health

These are some of the general rules of svarodaya for keeping the physical body and the subtle body in good health.

- The first basic rule regarding svarodaya is that a harmony should always be kept between the warm sun breath flowing through the right nadi and the cool breath of the left lunar nadi.
- During the bright half of the lunar month, the moon rules the night. Therefore, the effects of the sun are at a minimum. To harmonize this imbalance, it is necessary and advantageous to block the left nostril, and allow only the right channel to flow all night.
- Throughout the dark half of the month, the moon's influence is absent. So during this period, it is auspicious to block the sun channel and let the moon nadi flow all night.

- If at any time, and especially when out walking or exercising, you feel that your body temperature is suddenly increasing or you feel very tired, block the sun channel and let the vital breath flow through the moon nostril until the tiredness or the heat has gone.

- Vital energy can sometimes be lost through the ears as the two minor channels pusha and yashasvini connect the basic chakra with the ears. So when outdoors on a very hot or cold day, keep the ears covered.

- Meditation and visualization of the full moon resting on the area between the eyebrows is said to cure all psychosomatic illnesses and keep the mind calm and fresh. These benefits come only when one is capable of clear, complete visualization.

- When very thirsty and unable to get a drink, close the sun nadi and meditate on the tongue and the saliva dripping on to it. This will make it easier to endure the thirst.

- Some ancient texts on svarodaya suggest brisk, alternate-nostril breathing for about 2 minutes after each meal. This is said to help the subtle channels of the body to flow freely and the digestive organs to digest food.

- After having sexual intercourse in the manner suggested in the svarodaya texts, the couple should sip a lot of cool water.

PROLONGING GOOD HEALTH

Perform each of the three following basic ways of breathing for about 4 minutes every morning in order to have few illnesses and a healthy, long, and trouble-free life.

1. Breathe in and out through the nostrils.
2. Inhale through the mouth and exhale through the open nostril.
3. Breathe in through the open nostril and out through the mouth.

PROLONGING YOUTH WITH THE VIPARITA KARNI MUDRA

Those who have a desire to prolong their youth should frequently change the flow of the vital breath from one channel to the other. Besides this, they may attempt, under a yogi's guidance, the *viparita karni mudra* (inverted gesture) every morning and evening.

1. To perform the viparita karni mudra, first lie supine on a flat, hard surface and a woolen cloth.
2. Stretch your arms right above your head.
3. Now gently raise the legs together making an angle of 45° to the ground. The knees must be kept straight.

4. After achieving this, raise the legs further to make a 90° angle to the ground.

5. Now raise the buttocks and trunk by supporting the body with the palms held at the waist. In the final position, the body should be at an angle of 45° to the ground, with the legs held vertical.

6. Accompany this gesture with quick, forceful exhalations from the lungs. This mudra can be performed for about 10 to 20 seconds at a time. Many yogis can do this mudra for as long as 3 hours, but this is achieved only after long practice under a yogi-guru's instructions.

Specific Applications of Svarodaya for Good Health

Svarodaya also includes suggestions of remedies that can be applied for particular ailments.

Asthma Attack

When you feel an attack of asthma coming on, block your open nostril for 15 minutes. This will prevent the attack from getting serious. For long lasting relief keep this nostril blocked for at least a month.

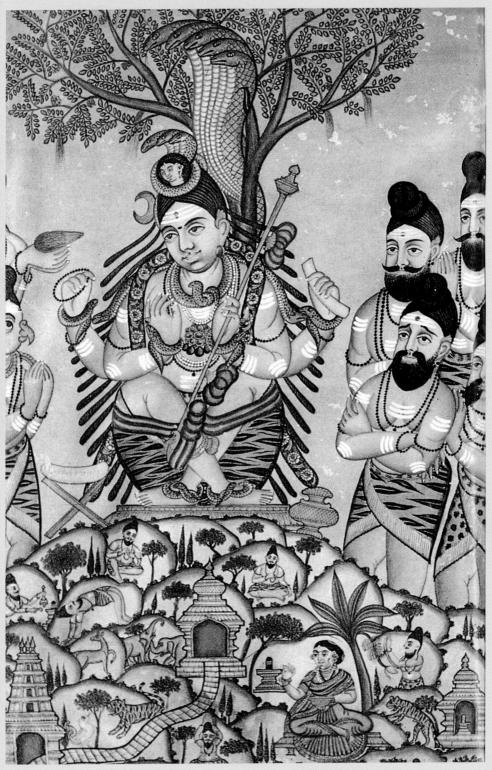

Plate 1. Shiva as Dakshinamurti (the southern image), representing the power of the intellect (buddhi). (Paper painting dated 1865; Mysore traditional style)

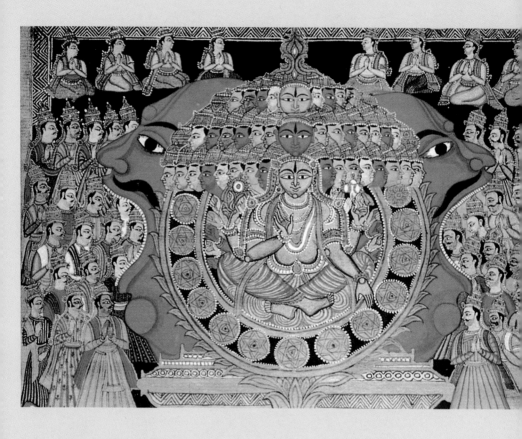

Plate 2. The all-manifesting and all-devouring cosmic form of the Lord. (Manuscript illustration from Srimad Bhagavad Gita; Mysore traditional style)

Plate 3 (right). Nadis of the subtle body spreading like veins through a pipal leaf. (Print of recent date, after the yoga-anka of Kalyan, a Hindi magazine)

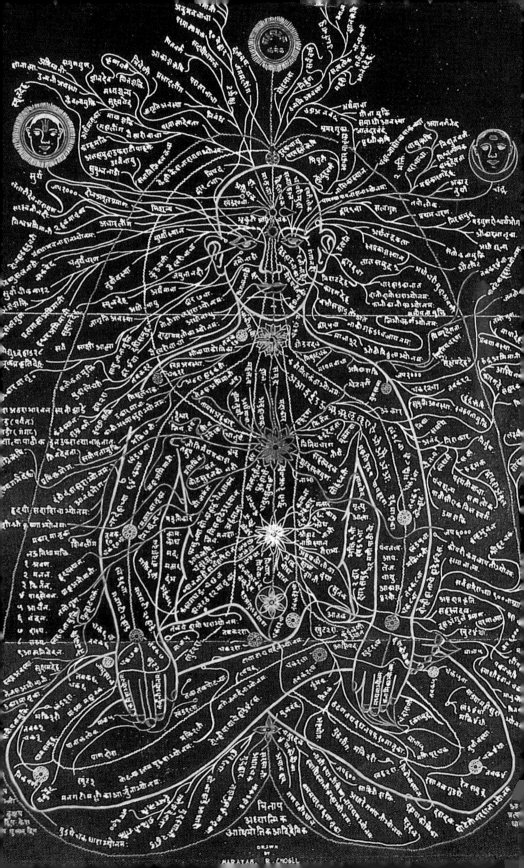

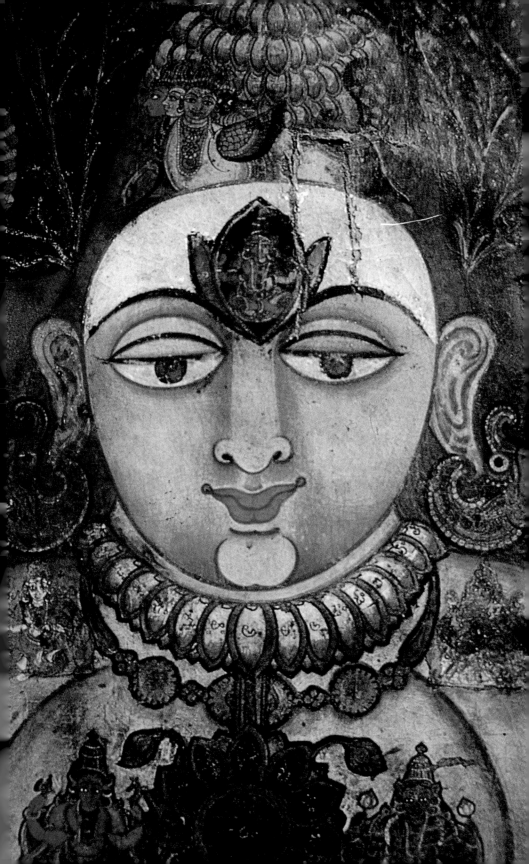

Plate 4 (left). Goddess Lakini, the power (Shakti) of the manipura chakra. (Nineteenth-century painting on board; Mysore traditional style)

Plate 5. The ajna chakra of enlightenment between the eyebrows. (Stone icon of the monkey god Hanuman with added glass eyes and gold foil)

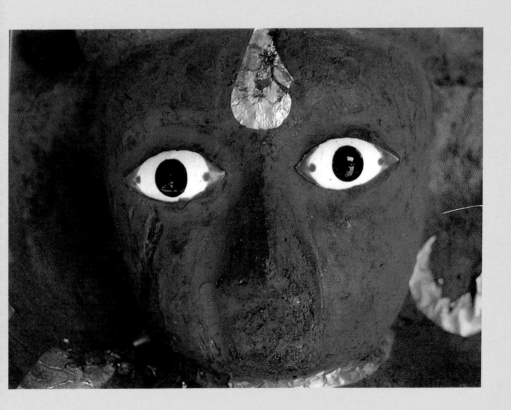

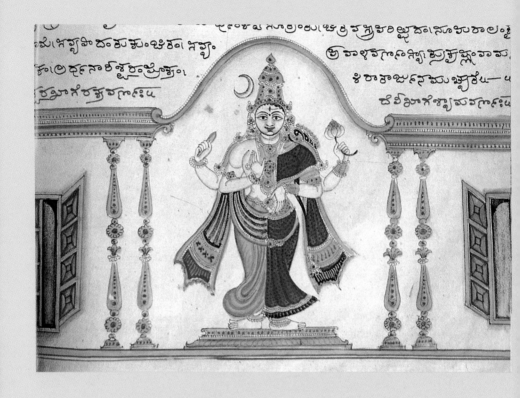

*Plate 6. Ardhanarishvara: Shiva as half male, half
female. (Manuscript painting from Sritattvanidhi of King
Mummadi Drisharaja Wadiyar III, 1799–1868; Mysore
traditional style)*

*Plate 7 (right). The three highest chakras and their
presiding deities (Eighteenth-century painting on cloth;
Mysore traditional style)*

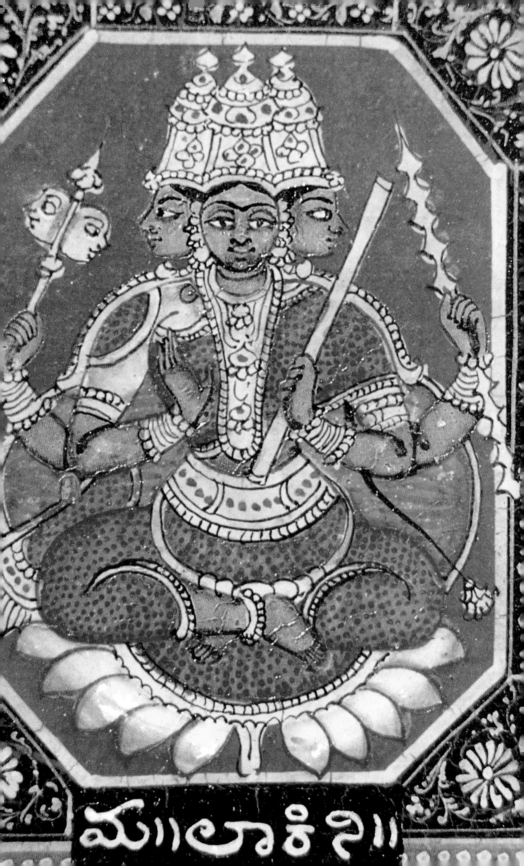

ಮಾಲಾಕಿ ಶಿ॥

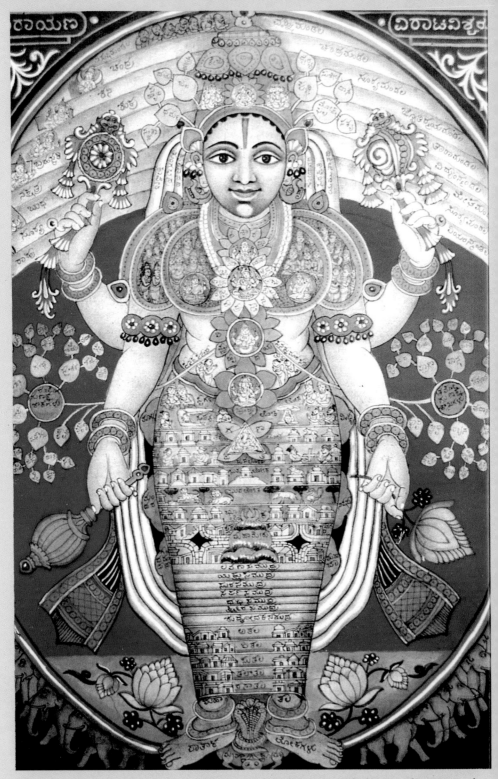

Plate 8. Adi-Narayana Virata Vishvarupa, showing various chakras in the universal or cosmic body. (Late nineteenth-century paper painting; Mysore traditional style)

Flatulence

For those who suffer from excess of gas in the intestine there is a very simple cure. About 15 minutes after every meal sit in the *virasana* (hero's posture) for 20 minutes. Virasana is formed in the same way as the vajrasana (see fig. 2.2 on page 56), except the heels are pressed against the outsides of the buttocks rather than placed underneath them.

Fever

If your body feels warm and feverish, block the open nostril. Keep it closed until you feel better again. You will find that the fever will go down very quickly, usually within a few hours.

Headache

For ordinary headaches lie flat and breathe deeply. Then get someone to tie a bandage around both elbows. The bandages should be tight enough to cause only a slight restriction in the circulation of blood. Untie the bandages after 4 minutes. If the headache still persists repeat this process as many times as necessary, offering a short break every 4 or 5 minutes to allow normal blood circulation to resume.

Those who suffer from persistent headaches should try the nose drinking method. Every morning, at sunrise, take a bowl full of cold water and try to suck some of it (at least about 2 spoonfuls) in through the open nostril. If this is done every morning, without a gap, for one month, your chronic headache will be cured forever.

If the headache is a migraine, tie a bandage around the left elbow if the pain is in the left side of the head; and around the right elbow if the pain is in the right side of the head. If the pain happens to be on the same side as the open nostril, block the nostril until the pain goes away.

Indigestion

Those who suffer from chronic indigestion should make it a point to eat only during the first 36 minutes of the flow of the sun channel. To cure indigestion quickly and permanently, sit in the padmasana posture for 10 minutes every morning.

Pain

For minor body pains, suddenly close and equally suddenly open the flowing nostril until the pain disappears. This opening and closing should be done rhythmically.

Spleen and Liver Troubles

If the spleen becomes enlarged due to jaundice or anemia, and if the liver is not functioning as well as it should, alternately contract and stretch your limbs for 5 minutes before you get out of bed every morning. Then shake your body from side to side for 10 minutes. This will help the spleen and liver to recover quickly and work much better.

Those who suffer from biliousness, skin rashes, and sores should perform the *shitali kumbhaka* (cold retention). This is done in the following manner: Sit in the siddhasana or padmasana posture. Protrude the tongue slightly out of the lips and breathe in through the mouth. Keep this air confined within the lungs for about 25 seconds, and then breathe out through the open nostril.

Weak Gums

If you have weak gums that make your teeth loose and painful, this is what you should do. While passing urine or excrement, clamp your jaws tightly together as if biting something very hard. Repeat this every day for two months and you will find a marked improvement in the health of your gums.

Reducing the Outflow of Vital Breath

Prana, the subtle vital energy that lives in the region of the heart, flows in and out with the physical breath. During normal breathing, the inhaled vital breath is 10 angulas long, while the exhaled breath is 12 angulas long. Thus we lose a lot of vital energy during daily respiration. This can shorten our life considerably. Typically, each cycle of exhalation and inhalation takes about 4 seconds to complete. The rate of respiration and the length of the vital breath is increased by physical action. For instance, eating increases the length of the vital breath to 18 angulas, walking to 20 angulas, running to 24 angulas, sexual intercourse to 60 angulas, and so on. If the rate of exhalation and inhalation is reduced and the flow of vital energy checked, we can easily increase our life span and gain control over our environment.

The benefits that can be derived from reducing the in and out flow of the vital breath are many.

1. If the outgoing breath is reduced to 11 angulas it is possible to gain control over the physical process of respiration.

2. If reduced to 10 angulas, one can achieve long-lasting peace of mind.

3. When diminished to 9 angulas, the individual is able to write spontaneous poetry and compose music.

4. Reduced to 8 angulas, one can attain clear diction and the ability to speak without hesitation or making mistakes.

5. If the vital breath is pared down to 7 angulas, the eyesight improves and one is able to see into the future.

6. When the outgoing vital breath is shortened down to 6 angulas, one becomes light and is able to fly like a hawk.

7. If further reduced to 5 angulas, one attains tremendous speed.

8. If decreased to 4 angulas, one attains the eight magical powers (siddhis) as well as the many minor siddhis.

The eight major siddhis are as follows:

- *Anima*—the ability to shrink to the size of an atom
- *Mahima*—to be able to increase in size according to desire
- *Garima*—to become extremely heavy
- *Laghima*—to become light and to levitate
- *Prati*—to bring anything within reach
- *Prakamya*—ability to immediately realize all desires
- *Vashitva*—the power to control all objects, animate and inanimate
- *Ishitva*—ability to create matter through the power of thought

The minor siddhis are also potent powers that can help in enjoying the world (*bhoga*) and experiencing spiritual bliss (*moksha*). They are:

- The power of subjugation (*vashikarana*)
- Magical eye salve or collyrium with which one can locate buried treasures (*gutikanjana*)
- Mastery in alchemy (*dhatuvada*)
- Power of destruction (*vidagdha*)
- Ability to stop fire (*agnistambhana*)
- Ability to stop floods (*jalastambhana*)
- Ability to stop speech (*vakstambhana*)
- Ability to fly in the air (*khecharitvam*)
- Ability to become invisible (*adrishyatvam*)
- Ability to attract another (*akarshanam*)
- Ability to influence young people (*yuva chitta vimohanam*)
- Ability to make the body beautiful and attractive (*nijanga saundaryam*)

9. When the outgoing vital breath is only 3 angulas, one becomes capable of finding the nine hidden treasures. According to ancient Indian occult tradition, the nine hidden treasures (*nava nidhi*) guarded by Lord Kubera are: tortoise (*kacchapa*), jasmine (*kunda*), delight (*nanda*), innumerable (*kharva*), crocodile (*makara*), sapphire (*nila*), conch (*shankha*), ruby (*padmaraga*), and the great lotus (*mahapadma*). Each of the nine treasures is under the care of a *yaksha* (mysterious one) appointed by their lord and master Kubera. The

theory is that the treasures lie buried deep inside the heart of the earth. They are, however, not inanimate things, but living treasures that can move from one place to another. They rarely come up to the surface of the earth. Only during the rule of a noble king do the nine treasures rise automatically to the earth's surface. It is said that a great yogi who has understood the secret science of the nine treasures (*nava nidhi vidya*) can attain them and make them rise. According to an oral tradition told to me by Swami Prakashananda, the nine treasures are really states of consciousness, which are attained by those who can stop the normal process of breathing and steady the mind.

10. If the exhaled vital breath is cut down to only 2 angulas, then the individual is able to change his physical shape at will. Tradition says that the Natha yogis were able to do this.

11. When the vital breath is diminished to 1 angula, one can easily become invisible and live in the subtle body for thousands of years.

12. Eventually, when the outgoing energy is so diminished that only a faint trace of the in/out flow remains, one will have reached immortality (*amaratvam*).

Predicting Death

The system of svarodaya shastra is frequently used to predict death. Describing this method may cause unnecessary anxiety to readers. Also, death does not always mean death of the physical body. The word is frequently used to symbolize spiritual illumination. Therefore, most of the methods of predicting death have been left out. Only the way of visualizing the shadow person (*chaya purusha*) is given here, as this has a wider meaning.

VISUALIZING THE SHADOW PERSON

To visualize the shadow person, find a deserted temple, or a burning ghat, or the bank of a river, or any other holy place unfrequented by people. Bathe in the river and sit on a kusha grass mat with your back to the rising sun. Steady your gaze on the neck of your own shadow. Do this for about two hours every day, for seven days. On the eighth day, while gazing at the shadow, recite the following mantra a hundred and eight times.

HRIM PARABRAHMANE NAMAH
(Hrim, I bow to the Transcendental Reality)

Then look up into the sky, and there you will see the chaya purusha—the form of your cosmic personality projected on to the sky.

If you see the shadow person as a complete, bright, and gray figure, it is auspicious and your yogic practices will be rewarded. You will eventually gain spiritual immortality. If the form of the shadow person is varicolored, you will attain all the eight occult powers. If the projected shadow person appears yellow, you will have to guard against illness. If a red shadow person is seen, your heart will be filled with fear in anticipation of future violence and aggression. But always remember that ill effects can be overcome with the inner guru's grace, with proper mantras, and with meditation. If the shadow person is dark black and its body appears mutilated, then either death or emancipation is near.

Divination

Many astrologers and yogis use the changing pattern of the vital breath for divination. They base their system on the correlation between their own flow of breath and the breath of the questioner. Some of the basic formulae on which they base their predictions are as follows:

- The left channel is generally more auspicious than the right.
- The breath of the earth and water elements is good; fire, air, and space elements are inauspicious.
- If the questioner stands or sits on the side of the diviner's open nostril, the answer should be favorable. The reverse of this is unlucky and the answer will be unfavorable.
- The flow of the central channel for long periods is generally considered to be inauspicious, with two exceptions: if the breath flowing from the central channel happens to be in the earth element on a Thursday, or if the breath is in the space element on a Saturday.

Some Questions and Their Answers

If asked whether a woman will become pregnant or not: if the inquirer is on the side of the diviner's closed nostril the answer should be "yes," otherwise "no."

If asked about the sex of an unborn child:

- Questioner's left channel and diviner's right channel flowing = short-lived male child
- Left channel of both flowing = long-lived male child
- Questioner's right channel and diviner's left channel flowing = short-lived female child

- Breath of both in the right channel = a beautiful girl who will live long

Questions about Travel

If the diviner's breath is in the moon nadi, and in one of the following elements, the results will be as follows:

- Earth element = happy and successful trip
- Water element = delay in reaching destination on account of floods
- Fire element = troublesome trip, beset with dangers
- Air element = unexpected delays and change of plans
- Space element = delay due to ill health

If the diviner's breath is in the sun nadi, then the fruits of the breath elements will be:

- Earth element = the trip will be successful and the traveler will return home happy
- Water element = traveler will find a happy and comfortable life in a foreign country and will not come home
- Fire element = the traveler will be in good health throughout the trip
- Air element = the traveler is likely to be delayed and may even get lost

• Space element = the traveler might have unexpected illness in the foreign country

Prediction of Battle Injuries

Some astrologers have even worked out a relationship between the breath elements and parts of the body likely to get hurt in a battle. Of course this applies to battles in the early days when men had only swords and spears to fight with. The correlation worked out by astrologers is as follows:

• Earth = abdomen
• Water = feet
• Fire = chest
• Air = thighs
• Space = head

Yearly Predictions

Yearly predictions based on the flow of vital breath should be made on the first day of the bright half of the month of Chaitra (March–April), or when the sun is moving southward (*dakshinayana*) from the summer to the winter solstice, or when the sun is moving northward (*uttarayana*) from the winter solstice.

If the moon appears at a time when the vital breath is flowing in the moon channel and is in the earth, water, or air element, the year will be prosperous, with plenty of rain and food. But if the breath is either in the fire or space element, there will be drought and famine. The central channel is always evil as far as mundane matters are concerned. If the sushumna is flowing at the time of the new moon, it foretells the coming of epidemics, wars, revolutions, and other such national calamities.

Predictions regarding the course of the coming year can also be made when the sun enters the sign of Aries (*Mesha samkramana* = vernal equinox). If on this day the breath is in the earth element, there will be adequate rainfall, fertile fields, plenty of food, and national expansion. The flow of the water element also stands for good rain and harvests. The fire element is generally unlucky, and its flow at the time of the vernal equinox denotes little or no rainfall throughout the year, and internal strife and setbacks in the country's economic development. The air element is also evil, and brings the well-known "six misfortunes" (*iti*): excessive rain in one part of the country, drought in another, locusts, rats, parrots that destroy fruits, and constant enemy invasions. The space element is the most inauspicious among all the five elements. It indicates the coming of a very miserable year.

If the breath that is flowing through the left nostril suddenly changes to the right nostril at the time of the vernal equinox, there will be wars throughout the country and the land will become like the lowest of all hells. The general rules used in predicting the course of the coming year apply equally when foretelling the course of a day or a month.

Attaining Liberation from the Cycle of Rebirth

The ida (left) is like the sacred river Ganga, the pingala (right) is like the Yamuna, and the central sushumna is the subterranean Sarasvati. The body through which these channels flow is like Prayaga (modern Allahabad), the king of holy cities. Just as the pilgrim who bathes at the confluence of the three sacred rivers is freed from all sins, similarly, the yogi who controls the flow of the three nadis gains freedom from the cycle of births and deaths and attains liberation (*mukti*).

Pranayama and the uddiyana bandha can be used to clean the impurities of the physical as well as the subtle body.

❀

BASIC PRANAYAMA

Sit in padmasana and perform pranayama as follows:

1. Puraka (filling): close the right nostril and inhale deeply through the left nostril.

2. Kumbhaka (retention): retain the inhaled air for as long as possible without discomfort.

3. Rechaka (expulsion): slowly exhale through the right nostril.

Repeat this process, using alternate nostrils, for as many times as you can without strain. Generally, the ratio of times between filling, retention, and expulsion is 1 : 4 : 2, but this can be changed a little for those who cannot retain the breath for too long on account of physical reasons.

The puraka is said to stabilize the body fluids and make the blood, the saliva, and the gastric juices flow freely. The kumbhaka prolongs life. Rechaka expels all impurities of the gross as well as the subtle body.

UDDIYANA BANDHA

After having mastered pranayama, attempt the uddiyana bandha (flying-up hold) to force the vital breath to fly up through the central nadi.

To perform the uddiyana bandha do the following:

1. Empty the lungs by a forceful expiration. When the lungs are empty, the diaphragm rises naturally into the thoracic cavity.

2. While the diaphragm is up, draw the intestines and the navel toward the back so that the abdomen rests against the back of the body, high up in the thorax. This can be done either sitting or standing. If done standing, place your hands firmly on the thighs, keep the legs apart, and bend your trunk slightly forward.

3. Maintain this posture for as long as you can hold the breath in without discomfort. The *bandha* can be done 5 to 8 times with short intervals.[1]

Once the vital breath starts flowing through the central sushumna nadi, it will result in samadhi, the final goal of all Yoga and meditation. In samadhi, the aspirant for liberation will experience Supreme Reality. The thousand-petaled lotus will open and the individual consciousness will unite with cosmic consciousness in final bliss.

❦

PURIFYING THE SUBTLE CHANNELS

Meditation on the area between the eyebrows (site of the ajna chakra and the optic thalamus) and the tip of the nose also helps in the purification of the subtle channels.

The method of this meditation is simple.

1. Find a quiet, clean spot and sit in either padmasana or any other comfortable posture.

2. Make sure that the vital breath is flowing in the auspicious channel for that particular day and time. If the breath is not in the auspicious nadi, change it using one of the methods described previously (see pages 48–49).

3. As soon as the vital breath starts flowing through the required channel, try to concentrate your sight on the tip of your nose. With both the eyes open, and the gaze pointed slightly downward, look at the tip of your nose. You will generally see only one side of the nose.

4. Take the visible side as the tip of the nose and meditate on it. This can be very tiring for the eyes, so practice this method for only 2 minutes at a time. It will take roughly two days before the eyes adjust to looking at such a near object. As soon as the eyes have adjusted, close them and concentrate on the mental image of the tip of the nose.

5. After a month or so, or as soon as you are able to meditate on the tip of the nose, lift the center of concentration upward until you reach the site of the ajna chakra. This also should be done with eyes closed by forming a mental image of the two-petaled lotus symbol of the ajna chakra.

The meditation method given in step 4 is known as

bhuchari (earth-pointing) and in step 5 as *khechari* (sky-pointing). Once the bhuchari and khechari meditations have been perfected, the inner sight will become restless and unsteady. This is called *chachari* (moving) and heralds the coming of the final stage of *agochari,* when the object of concentration vanishes and the mind is completely absorbed into the Infinite. When this stage is reached, the vital breath begins to flow through the central channel and the meditator becomes enlightened.

Most traditional works on the svarodaya shastra stress the need for secrecy. The reason for this, according to the Shiva Svarodaya Shastra, is that many charlatans and so-called gurus may try to use the knowledge to gain wealth and to harm others. A true yogi, on the other hand, will not be tempted by selfish ends and will have no need to impress the crowds. He or she will know that the way to spiritual freedom is not cleared by performing miracles.

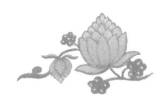

Chapter Four

TANTRIK AND YOGIC PRACTICES FOR LIBERATION

Consciousness

According to yogic tradition, there are four states of human consciousness. The most basic and exoteric is the waking state, or *jagriti*. Then comes the state of dreams, or *svapna*, when there is no awareness of the outside world, but the mind is not at rest. The worlds of the subconscious and the superconscious are active. The third state is that of deep, dreamless sleep, or *sushupti*, when the mind is apparently at rest, but the seed of all mental activities lies dormant. As soon as the individual awakens, and the mind goes into the waking state, the dormant seed sprouts again into the many manifestations of the mind. The fourth state of *turiya* is not an ordinary one. It is the state when the mind has gone and there is no longer a sense of "I-ness."

Tantra and Yoga offer a variety of practices (*sadhana*) that lead the individual mind to be absorbed into the universal mind, a few of which are given here.

Soham Sadhana

As mentioned earlier, breathing, both physical and subtle, is made up of two acts: inspiration, in which the air is taken into the lungs; and expiration, in which the inspired air is driven out of the lungs. The air that is driven out of the lungs makes the sound *ham;* and the inhaled air produces the sound *sah.* The two sounds together make the Sanskrit word *hamsah* (literally "goose"), which is a synonym for the Supreme Spirit.

In Indian mythology, the goose is a bird that can separate milk from water, a normally impossible task. This special ability of the mythical goose has made it a symbol of discrimination (*viveka*) between what is real (the spirit) and what is merely transient (the world of names and forms). Moreover, the goose is pure white and spotless and therefore said to represent the soul.

The *ham* sound symbolizes the male creative principle of consciousness and is known as the seed mantra of Shiva. The *sah* sound represents the female creative principle of energy and is the seed mantra of Shakti. When the word *hamsa* is reversed, it spells *soham* in Sanskrit. The word *soham* is the famous Upanishadic statement (*mahavakya*) stressing the identity of the individual soul (*aham* = I) and the Supreme Spirit (*sah* = That) (see Isha Upanishad, 16).

The word *soham* is made up of the following vowels and consonants: *s + o + h + a + m.* When the consonants *s* and *h* are taken away from *soham* we are left with OM, the greatest of all mantras (thought forms). This sacred mantra covers the entire range of articulate sound, and is therefore the symbol of the cosmic order as understood by the human mind.

At a practical level, the *soham* sound that the inhaled and exhaled breaths make can be used as a means of developing awareness. This is traditionally called the practice of spontaneous repetition (*ajapa japa*) and is very effective in cultivating awareness and controlling the mind. This technique is also known in Buddhism as the mindfulness of breathing (*anapanassati vipassana*). The soham japa is a natural method (*sahaja*) because no mantras, no *mala* (rosary), and no initiation are needed. All that is required is to be constantly aware of the two sounds made by the in and out acts of respiration. The sound is always with us, and remains constant during all states of consciousness: waking, dreaming, and deep sleep. If an awareness of the *soham* sound can be kept going through the three states of consciousness, then the individual reaches the fourth state of enlightenment.

At first, however, it is difficult to be continuously aware of the *soham* sound. For this, a little formal and preliminary practice (*sadhana*) is necessary.

ॐ

PRACTICING AWARENESS OF THE SOHAM SOUND

Choose a clean place, free from noise and other distur-
bances. The place should be without any unpleasant associations. A naturally beautiful place near a flowing stream
or in a grove of flowering trees would be ideal. It can be
any time of the day or night. What is important is that the
mind should be calm and relaxed.

1. To begin with, sit in any comfortable posture, with the
   eyes either closed or open, as convenient.

2. Then breathe in slowly and try to hear the *so* sound. If at
   first you do not hear the sound, try to either imagine it
   or mentally repeat it.

3. While breathing out, the *ham* sound can also be heard,
   imagined, or mentally repeated. Care should be taken
   to see that the breathing is continuous and the *soham* is
   not broken up like a verbal mantra.

Generally, when one becomes conscious of the process
of breathing, its rate alters a little. This can become uncom-
fortable. If this happens, rest a little and then resume the
practice. Ten to fifteen minutes at the beginning should
become longer and longer until the awareness of the sound
becomes natural and spontaneous. When this happens

one might feel that the breath has stopped. But there is no need to worry as this is a sign that the practice has now become natural. This is the *sahaja* state.

The sahaja state leads to total awareness of breathing; with the awareness of breathing comes an awareness of the nature of emotional, psychological, and physical conditioning. When you are aware of the nature of conditioning of the mind you are free from the bonds of attachment. In freedom is the final meeting of consciousness (Purusha) and energy (Prakriti).

Color Meditation (Varna Dhyana)

Color meditation is generally considered helpful in maintaining inner calm and in understanding the subtle working of the vital energies of the human body. It is essential to remember that the color meditation is directed toward emotions, and so it is necessary to understand the significance of the colors.

The first color for meditation is red. This color represents all the fiery emotions like anger, passion, lust, hate, violence, and constant activity. The purpose of meditating on this color is to become one with the emotions it symbolizes, and to understand these emotions in our psychological makeup. In Indian mythology, red is associated with

Brahma, the principle of creation, and the mother goddess, the basic energy of the cosmos.

The second color for meditation is black. This symbolizes all the negative feelings of the human mind. Depression, sorrow, grief, and so on, are all referred to as "dark" emotions. Negative attitudes and emotions are harmful to our physical and mental health. But to overcome them, we must understand them. And to understand them we must accept them. We generally try to push the negative part of ourselves into the subconscious and project only the good. But merely repressing the negative aspects does not make us free from them. They have to be brought into the open and understood. Any power that is understood loses its dangerous quality. Meditation on the color black helps us in bringing the dark part of our mind to the surface. Black is a symbol of night, sleep, and death, and hence represents Lord Shiva, the universal power of death.

Having understood and gone beyond the disturbing emotions of passion (rajas = red) and negativity (tamas = black), meditate upon white, the color of inner peace and harmony. This is the symbol of Lord Vishnu, the cosmic principle of order and balance. White also represents light and wisdom, and stands for purity (sattva).

❧

COLOR MEDITATION

The method of color meditation is simple.

1. Sit in a comfortable posture. Generally padmasana or *sukhasana* (easy posture) is recommended, but any posture will do.

2. Then take a large piece of cloth or paper of the required color. Stare at the colored cloth or paper and allow the color to become part of you. Let your entire body take on the color you are meditating upon.

3. When you feel that the color has covered you completely with its nature, close your eyes and visualize the color inside you.

When you can successfully visualize the color with your eyes closed, you have perfected color meditation. The various physical and psychic benefits will come automatically to you.

Meditation on the Five Elements

Meditation on the five elements (*pancha mahabhutas*) is commended in the Tantras. It is said that this form of meditation frees the mind from the usual narrow concerns and gives it a sense of its vast potential powers. The human mind is capable of enormous creativity, but unfortunately most of us are so engrossed in petty, everyday concerns that we have no time to comprehend our hidden potential. Meditation on the natural elements shows us how we are a part of this universe and how we share all the powers of the cosmos.

❀

ELEMENT MEDITATION

The laya yoga method of meditation on the elements begins with sitting in a comfortable posture and then imagining that the body and mind are becoming one with the elements. Usually the most gross element is taken first, and the mind is gradually allowed to move to the more subtle elements until finally it is absorbed into the most subtle element of all: space. As the element meditation moves upward through the body, each element is associated with a color, shape, and deity, which reveal their universal dimensions.

Earth

The first element is earth (prithvi). This is the basic material from which our bodies are made, and we live on its most gross and solid form. Symbolically the earth represents stability and volume and is therefore shown as a yellow square and is ruled by the lord of cosmic evolution, Brahma. In our bodies, the influence of earth extends from the feet to the knees.

1. To meditate on the earth element, sit absolutely motionless and try to visualize the entire planet Earth as being a part of your body.

2. Gradually identify the different parts of the body with the various features of Earth. The streams and rivers are the blood vessels, the forest trees are the hairs on the body, and so on.

3. When you feel that your body has lost its individuality and has become this entire planet Earth, then move on to the next element.

Water

The second element for meditation is water (ap). It is not just the water we see in lakes, rivers, and the sea, but all flowing things. All that is capable of change and can flow has the spirit of water in it. Water is symbolized as a white circle: white because all colors are contained in it; and circular because it represents flow, a return to the source, and rhythm.

The human body from the knees to the navel is ruled

by water, and its ruling deity is Lord Narayana, the power of perpetual life. The word *narayana* also means "moving on water," and this may be a symbolic reference to the fact that life originated in water, and it still begins in the amniotic fluid that surrounds the embryo. Let your mind and body dwell upon the flow of water, and gradually they will lose their definite shapes and melt away into the rhythms of the universe.

Fire

When the mind and body have become liquid, change to the next element, fire (agni). The rule of fire extends from the navel to the heart, and is represented by a red triangle pointing upward to signify its vertical movement. Meditation on fire just after meditating on water brings about a balance. The cool and liquid nature of the mind is now transformed into heat and activity. The lord of tears and death, Rudra, rules this element.

1. To meditate on fire allow your mind and body to feel the heat rising from the navel to the heart center.

2. As you progress in the identification of your body and mind with fire, the body temperature will rise.

3. When the body becomes too hot for comfort, change your meditation to the next element, air (vayu).

Air

Air governs the body from the heart to the area between the eyebrows. It is symbolized as a black or blue crescent and is ruled by Ishvara, the lord of the cosmos. The first three elements have form, but air is formless and therefore more subtle. Meditation on air brings the mind closer to the formless reality, which is the goal of all spiritual life.

1. At first let your body be fanned by the refreshing air.

2. Then imagine that your mind has become very very subtle.

3. Allow your body to lose its gross form and become as light as air. You will feel that you are actually levitating.

Air is also the vehicle of the vital energies, so meditation on it will quickly lead you to the final stage of meditation on the elements: the stage of the most subtle, space (akasha).

Akasha

The space element rules the area above the eyebrows and extends beyond the limits of the human body into space. As space is beyond all human senses, it has no symbolic shape or color. Sometimes, however, it is represented as a point (bindu) to stress the idea that it stands on the threshold of the manifest and the unmanifest, the seen and the unseen, the gross and the subtle, and all other such dualities.

When the mind is completely identified with the space element in meditation, it is "no more." This is enlightenment, the final goal of spiritual sadhana. The space element is traditionally ruled by Sadashiva (always auspicious), an aspect of Shiva.*

Accompanying Meditation with a Mantra

All the meditations so far described can be accompanied with the repetition of a mantra (*mantra japa*). This helps concentration, because constant repetition of a set of sounds induces a mild state of autohypnosis and calms the restless mind. A mantra is a sound pattern that can either be a name of a deity, a monosyllable like OM, a Sanskrit phoneme imitating a natural sound, or a short prayer.

The most gross stage in the formation of a mantra sound

---

*Sadashiva is the presiding deity of the vishuddha chakra and also the third tattva coming from Shiva (as the ultimate Reality) in the evolutionary scheme. Sadashiva is also a philosophical concept in the texts of Kashmir Shaivism of the Trika school. God in the form of pure knowledge is called Shiva, and in the form of energy and action is known as Shakti. When these two are in balance, this state of being is known as Maheshvara. According to monistic theory of Shaivism, as given in the Shiva-mahapurana (Rudra samhita), after the time of the great dissolution, when all things were destroyed, there arose creative energy called Sadashiva.[1]

pattern is the sound uttered aloud with the help of the vocal cords, the lips, the tongue and the teeth. This is called "the audible mantra," or *vaikhari*. Before audible sound can be produced, there is a stage when the speech centers in the brain activate the vocal apparatus. No audible sound has yet been produced, but the form that the pronounced sound will take is already formulated clearly in the mind. There is no sound but only mentation. This stage is called "the intermediate," or *madhyama*. The basic human potential to be able to arrange sounds into meaningful speech is called "the foreseen," or *pashyanti,* in the Tantras. The center of the pashyanti stage of sound is said to be in the anahata chakra (cardiac plexus or heart chakra). Pure sound, as a form of kinetic energy that can become manifest as soon as there is vibration, is called "the beyond," or *para,* stage of sound.

In the Tantras the four states of human consciousness are compared to the four stages of sound: *jagriti* (waking state) = vaikhari, *svapna* (dream state) = madhyama, *sushupti* (deep sleep state) = pashyanti, and *turiya* (the "fourth," pure consciousness) = para. The practice of meditation and mantra japa based on the four states/stages tries to lead the mind from the gross to the subtle and beyond. This process of absorbing the human mind into the universal mind is also called laya yoga.

When a mantra is repeated aloud it is said to be at the

gross, audible stage of vaikhari. Most mantras are at this stage. But when a serious disciple repeats a mantra silently—when the lips and the tongue move but no audible sound is produced—the mantra is said to be in the madhyama stage. When the mind has become silent and the mantra becomes automatic and goes on like the movement of the breath, it has reached the stage of pashyanti. Beyond pashyanti, the mantra, along with the disciple's mind, merges with the Infinite. This is the para stage of the mantra. It is said in the Taittiriya Upanishad (II, 9):

> He who knows the bliss of Brahman, whence words and the mind turn away and are unable to reach it, he is not afraid of anything.

Magical Powers

With practice, control over each chakra of the subtle body can be achieved. As the yogi attains power over one chakra after another, he or she will find that magical powers are acquired along with psychic experiences.

Control over the first chakra and its element earth gives the ability to make the body as light as air for astral travel and levitation and to shine with a golden aura. The second chakra and its element water gives the power to live for long periods without food or water, to survive under water, and to make the body shine with a silver aura. The control over fire, the element of the third chakra, confers the ability to eat enormous amounts of food without bad effects, to endure strong heat, and to make the body shine with a red aura. Command over air and its chakra in the subtle body gives the capacity to fly like birds and to understand their language. The space element invests the yogi with the fantastic capacity to look into, beyond, and before time as well as the eight famed magical powers (siddhis) mentioned earlier. Another list and interpretation of the eight magical or occult powers is given in some hatha yoga texts. According to them:

- Anima (atomization) enables the yogi to become infinitely small in order to understand the inner nature of atoms and molecules that form the building blocks of this universe. This power can be gained by deep meditation on the heart center.
- Mahima is just the opposite, and allows the siddha to become vast, so as to be able to see the cosmic structure of stars and galaxies and penetrate beyond space and time to experience the ultimate Reality. This power can be gained by meditating on the essence of the intellect (mahat), the first transformation of the primeval state of nature (Prakriti).

- Garima is the capacity to acquire enormous weight, which leads to permanence and stability. Constant meditation on the earth element is said to confer this power.

- Laghima is the power to become light, leave the body at will, and do astral projection. Deep meditation on, and identification with, the element air is the origin of this siddhi.

- Prakamya is to develop an irresistible will that can compel others to obey one's wishes. Meditation on the space element leads to this siddhi, and the ability to hypnotize is a form of this power.

- Ishitva is the power to control nature, to stop the wind, rain, storms, fire, and earthquakes. One may look upon the marvels of modern science and technology as mild examples of this siddhi.

- Vashitva is the ability to control animate nature and to influence the behavior of men and animals. Both ishitva and vashitva are gained by meditation on the creative power of the universe.

- *Kamavashayitvam* allows the yogi to take any form at will and to fulfill all desires. This power is attained by meditating on the principle of primeval ego (ahamkara) and is quite common. One frequently hears of saints and religious leaders who can feed thousands of devotees on just a pot of rice.

These magical powers, and many other sub-siddhis that come along with them, are by-products of yogic discipline. When the various stages of yoga are perfected and one goes deeper into meditation, the eight occult powers come naturally. They are symbols of spiritual progress. Although they are called "magical" and "occult," they are in fact only highly developed and perfected aspects of the energies of the human mind: the energy of vision (*jnana shakti*), of will (*iccha shakti*), and of action (*kriya shakti*).[2]

The true achievement is not to get carried away with these powers but to go beyond them to ultimate enlightenment. However, some yogis, who are not interested in the "ultimate" but value material benefits more than spiritual ones, use these powers for selfish reasons. For such people they can become impediments on the spiritual path. This is because if one uses siddhis, one is bound to attract a lot of attention and become famous. Fame generally leads to pride, and pride is the greatest obstacle to inner growth.

A true siddha yogi who has established complete control over his or her nervous system, subtle body, and the various states of consciousness has neither the will nor the need to use any of the magical powers attained. If they are used at all, it is only for compassionate reasons. All such a person really desires is to be united forever with the Supreme Reality.

OM tat sat (OM that alone is)

NOTES

Chapter One

1. The Diagram Group, *The Brain: A User's Manual* (London: New English Library, 1982), 460–77.

2. Vijayendra Pratap, "Diurnal Pattern of Nostril Breathing—An Exploratory Study," *Yoga-Mimamsa* 14: 3, 4, (1971–72): 1–17.

3. M. V. Bhole and P. V. Karambelkar, "Significance of Nostrils in Breathing," *Yoga-Mimamsa* 10:4 (1968): 1–12.

4. S. Rao and A. Potdar, "Nasal Airflow with Body in Various Positions," *Journal of Applied Physiology* 28:2 (1970): 162–65.

5. James Funderburk, *Science Studies Yoga: A Review of Physiological Data* (Honesdale, Pa.: Himalayan International Institute of Yoga Science and Philosophy of the U.S.A., 1977), 48–50.

6. Robert Ornstein, *The Psychology of Consciousness* (New York: Penguin Books, 1986).

7. Arthur Avalon (Sir John Woodroffe), *The Serpent Power: Being the Satcakranirupana and Padukapancaka* (Calcutta-London: Tantrik Texts II, 1913).

Chapter Three

1. Swami Vishnudevananda, *The Complete Illustrated Book of Yoga* (New York: Pocket Books, 1972), 42; and Hatha Yoga Pradipika, chapter III, verses 57–58.

Chapter Four

1. For more details on Sadashiva see Surendranath Dasgupta, *A History of Indian Philosophy,* vol. V, rep. ed. (Delhi: Motilal Barnarsidass, 1975). Originally published in 1922.
2. Alain Daniélou, *While the Gods Play* (Rochester, Vt.: Inner Traditions, 1987), 94–96.

BIBLIOGRAPHY

Chaplin, J. P. *Dictionary of the Occult and Paranormal*. New York: Dell Publishing Co., 1976.

Daniélou, Alain. *Hindu Polytheism*. London: Routledge & Kegan Paul, 1964.

——. *While the Gods Play*. Rochester, Vt.: Inner Traditions, 1987.

Diagram Group, The. *The Brain: A User's Manual*. London: New English Library, 1982.

Eliade, Mircea. *Yoga: Immortality and Freedom*. Princeton, N.J.: Bollingen Series, LVI, 1969.

Funderburk, James. *Science Studies Yoga: A Review of Physiological Data*. Honesdale, Pa.: Himalayan International Institute of Yoga Science and Philosophy of the U.S.A., 1977.

Iyengar, B. K. S. *Light on Pranayama*. London: George Allen & Unwin, 1981.

Raman, B. V. *A Manual of Hindu Astrology*. Bangalore: India Book House, 1979.

"Sadhana Anka," *Kalyan* 15 (1940). [Note: The *Kalyan* is a monthly magazine published in Hindi by Gita Press in Gorakhpur, India. Gita Press also publishes a monthly English language magazine, the *Kalyana-Kalpataru*.]

Sharma, N. N. *Yoga Karnika of Nath Aghorananda*. Delhi: Eastern Book Linkers, 1981.

Vaidya, S. M. *Pranavopasana* (Marathi). Bombay: Tukaram Book Depot, 1975.

Velenkar, Sharad, *Siva Svarodaya Shastra* (Sanskrit text and Marathi translation). Bombay: Institute of Parapsychology, 1979.

Vishnudevananda, Swami. *The Complete Illustrated Book of Yoga.* New York: Pocket Books, 1972.

Walker, Benjamin. *Encyclopaedia of Esoteric Man.* London: Routledge & Kegan Paul, 1977.

Yoga: An Instruction Booklet. Madras, India: Vivekananda Kendra Publications, 1982.

INDEX

Page numbers in *italic* refer to illustrations.

Kubera, Lord, 94–95
kuhu, 24
kumbhaka, 7–8
kundalini, 29, 31, 36–38
kurma, 25

laghima, 93, 124
Lakini, pl.4, 31
lalana, 33–34
laya yoga, 56
liberation, 102–6
lingam, 29, 35
liver troubles, 90–91
lokas, 38–39
Lord, pl.2

madhyama, 121
magical powers, 122–25
mahabhutas, 20, *21*
maha shunya, 34
mahat, 19, *21*
mahima, 93, 123
manas, 19–20
manas chakra, 35
manas loka, 38
manipura chakra, pl.4, 31–32
mantras, 28, 120–22
Matsyendranatha, 18
meditation, 28
Mercury, 46
meru danda, 26
mind. *See* manas
moksha, 93
movement. *See* rajas

mudras, 36–38
mula bandha, 37
muladhara chakra, 23, 29, 31

nadis, pl.3, 23–25, 27–29, *64–65*
nadi shodhana, 27
naga, 25
nakshatras, 61
natha, 18
Natha sect, 18
nauli, 28
neti, 27
nine hidden treasures, 94–95
nirguna, 43
nirmanu, 27
niyama, 7
nostrils, 11, 14–17, 43–44
nourishment distribution. *See*
    dhananjaya

occult, 5–6
OM, 58, 110, 120
Omkara, 35
organs of action. *See* karma
    indriyas

padmasana, 8–10, *9*
pain, 90
pancha mahabhutas, 115–20
panchangas, 45–46
pancha pranas, 24
Parvati, 17–18, 35, 36
pashyanti, 121
pingala, 24, 25–28, 43

Books of Related Interest

Breath, Mind, and Consciousness
by Harish Johari

Tools for Tantra
by Harish Johari

Chakras
Energy Centers of Transformation
by Harish Johari

Microchakras
Techniques for InnerTuning
by Sri Shyamji Bhatnagar and David Isaacs, Ph.D.

Breathing
Expanding Your Power and Energy
by Michael Sky

Ways to Better Breathing
by Carola Speads

The Yoga of Truth
Jnana: The Ancient Path of Silent Knowledge
by Peter Marchand

Yoga Spandakarika
The Sacred Texts at the Origins of Tantra
by Daniel Odier

INNER TRADITIONS • BEAR & COMPANY
P.O. Box 388
Rochester, VT 05767
1-800-246-8648
www.InnerTraditions.com

Or contact your local bookseller